The Medical Practitioner's Survival Handbook

by Jon Hultman, DPM, MBA

MEDICAL BUSINESS ADVISORS PUBLISHING
Los Angeles, California

Limits of Liability and Disclosure of Warranty
The Author and Publisher of this book have used their best efforts in preparing the book in order to provide accurate and current information. This book should not be used as a substitute for competent legal advice regarding any material presented which might be subject to local, state, and federal regulations. The Author and Publisher make no warranty of any kind, expressed or implied, with regard to the material presented within the book.

Editor: Luke Hultman
Associate Editor: Patricia Hultman
Artwork: Emily Hultman

Printed in the United States of America

Medical Business Advisors, Publisher, Los Angeles, CA 90025

Table of Contents

Chapter 1

Know Your Costs

Chapter 2

Use Leverage to Your Advantage

Chapter 3

Think Like an Engineer

Chapter 4

Satisfy Your Customers

Chapter 5

Retain a Smart and Loyal Staff

Chapter 6

Fix Your Scheduling Process

Chapter 7

Get the Most Out of Your EMR

Chapter 8

Increase the Size of Your Practice

Chapter 9
Eliminate Psychological Barriers to Practice Improvement

Chapter 10
Know the Value of Your Practice

Chapter 11

Be Smarter with Your Money

Preface

My first book, Reengineering the Medical Practice, was published by St. Anthony's in 1994. As it happens, the environment physicians face today – seventeen years later – is strikingly similar to the one we faced then. Fortunately, the principles and strategies discussed in the reengineering book have withstood the test of time and have resulted in increased quality, lower costs, and improved medical practice performance for its readers. These same principles lay the foundation for material discussed in The Medical Practitioner's Survival Handbook.

Whether you practice solo, in a small group, as part of a large network, or in a "supergroup," the same laws of science encountered in your pre-med education can be applied in unique, innovative ways to your medical practice. They will help you to increase quality and productivity while decreasing costs. These strategies make sense in any healthcare environment, but in the current high volume, price competitive market in which payers and employers are seeking to reward efficiency and quality, the potential opportunities to be gained through application of these principles are signifiant. Given the similarity of the 1994 medical arena to that of 2011, I feel that the preface taken from the reengineering book applies as well today as it did seventeen years ago.

Preface from Reengineering the Medical Practice, 1994

Let's face it, medicine is a business, and that business is changing fast, very, very fast. The "tried and true" isn't working today, and by tomorrow, it will fail completely. In this competitive climate, lower reimbursement rates and higher costs have combined to reduce profitability and quality of care. To survive, you will need tools that will help you compete profitably and avoid costly mistakes.

The good news is that addressing these problems is not a mysterious proposition. It will, however, require a change in the way you do things. Other industries experiencing similar competitive environments have adapted successfully. The bad news is that while major industries have made this transition, many corporations competing within those industries have failed along the way. This is why Reengineering the Medical Practice was written. The same sound business practices employed by businesses that succeeded in the corporate arena can be adapted to work in your medical office or clinic. As the practice of medicine and the entire health care industry change, the skills that have worked so well for you in the past must be augmented with business skills designed to increase quality, improve efficiency, and lower costs. This book will provide you with the business knowledge needed to bridge the gap between today's and tomorrow's practice of medicine.

In every industry, the most successful companies are those which make the most profit. The highest profits are achieved by those with the capability to adapt to change and deliver, in the least costly way, a high volume of those quality features most valued by customers. To understand the type of change necessary for adapting, consider a problem that Ford Motor Company faced in the early 1980s. Ford employed more than 500 people in accounts payable and realized that it needed to cut costs in this department in order to better compete against foreign imports. To address this inefficient process, Ford planned to install a new computer system with the hope of reducing its accounts payable head count by 20 per cent. Compare Ford's hoped for outcome to the reality of Mazda's accounts payable department which, during this same time period, employed only five people! Obviously, Mazda's accounts payable process was not simply an improved version of Ford's; it was an entirely different "species" that had been accomplished through workflow analysis and process re-engineering. Given the fact that all value delivered by medicine is achieved through some type of "process," similar opportunities for improvement are substantial.

This book represents the results of two decades of analysis and study of the successful principles utilized by other industries that have already been through the same competitive changes that medicine is currently experiencing. It adapts those same principles for use in attacking the cost, quality, access, and profitability problems currently faced by physicians. The relevant information needed to succeed in a price competitive market is included in this book, and the business disciplines needed to understand and effectively apply these concepts are presented in a language understandable to physicians.

Chapter 1

Know Your Costs

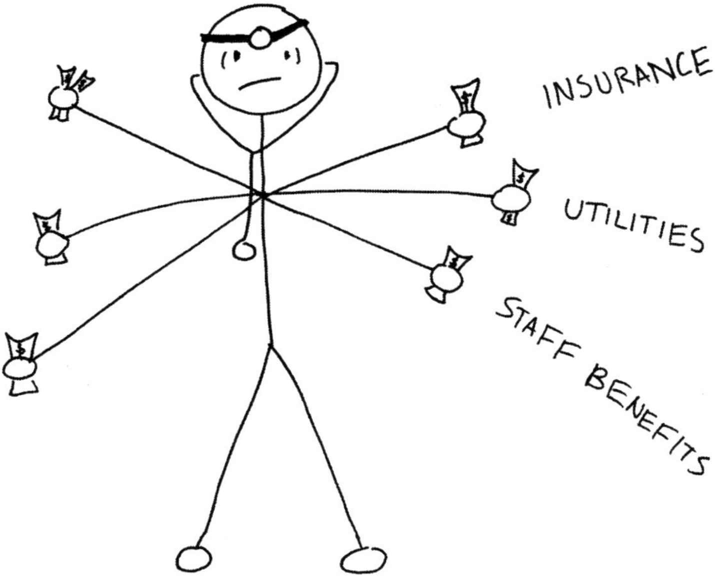

Revenue and Costs

We've all heard the saying, "It's not how much you make that counts, it's how much you keep." Let us consider this in terms of the medical practice. Although top line revenue for today's typical practice remains relatively high, the amount that drops to the bottom line as profit continues to shrink. This is partly due to lower fees, but doctors today are facing even bigger challenges – high patient volumes and more complex business operations – resulting in overly high costs. These circumstances have propelled the understanding and effective application of efficiency concepts to the forefront of the tools a practitioner must wield in order to achieve ultimate success. As we will see throughout this book, efficiency has a positive impact on quality as well as on profitability; a doctor who focuses on "quality" through efficiency will achieve more profit in the process.

In business, profit results from supplying a product or service that a customer values and is willing to pay more for than it costs to produce. Profit is important to the success of every business and is a reflection of its value. Unnecessary costs can significantly reduce this "value" – sometimes to the point that the business ceases to exist. Before analyzing the business operational areas that impact quality and profit, it is important that we first understand profit from a financial perspective, starting with the profit equation.

The Profit Equation

Profit is defined as revenue minus cost, and revenue is defined as price times volume. Combining these two equations, we arrive at the formula:

Profit = (Price ∗ Volume) – Cost

In a price competitive market, price is often out of our control and is certain to decrease. Volume is out of our direct control and could move either up or down. The only part of the equation under our direct control is cost. Our profit equation reveals that an increase in volume, a decrease in cost, or the combination of both, could offset a decline in profit resulting from lower prices. The following is the “winning” strategy when price is declining:

$$\textbf{Profit} = (\textbf{Price}\downarrow * \textbf{Volume}\uparrow) - \textbf{Cost}\downarrow$$

Since volume is not under our direct control, it may decline, and if it does, costs must be aggressively reduced in order to offset this decline and, thereby, maintain or increase profit. While practitioners fear the possibility of failure resulting from an inability to secure contracts that pay reasonable fees, they should also be aware that failure can be caused by obtaining contracts that, while they increase volume, cause costs to increase at a faster rate than revenue. Any strategy that ignores costs is a “losing” one, one that will result in lower profit.

Cutting costs should not be simply a matter of spending less or “doing without.” In a medical practice, this type of cost-cutting results in lower quality – especially when patient volume is increasing. The key to success is maintaining, or increasing, quality while simultaneously increasing volume and decreasing costs. This process is not an easy one but is made possible through implementation of efficiency improvements. Efficiency techniques and the tools for their successful implementation will be discussed throughout this book.

Cost Trends Over Time

Over the lifetime of a business, costs tend to follow a “U” shaped curve. At first, they decrease rapidly as volume increases. This is an intuitive concept, and most people understand this relationship as being related to cost-savings resulting from *economies of scale*. If a practice’s annual overhead is $250,000 and only one patient is treated, the total cost of treating that one patient is $250,000. When a second patient is treated, the cost decreases to $125,000 per patient; adding just one patient cuts costs-per-patient in half. When 1,000 patients are treated, the average cost is $250 per patient. At this point, treating one more patient (patient number 1,001) reduces costs by only $00.25 per patient. As you can see, cost per patient continues to decline at this point, but at a much slower rate.

Increasing volume helps to reduce costs by spreading overhead over a greater number of patients; however, there are also some new costs associated with any increase in patient volume. With each additional patient, a small, incremental cost related to supplies is incurred, and when a pivotal number of patients is reached, additional personnel may be required to deal with the higher volume. At this point, any additional increase in volume may raise costs enough to actually lower profit. As patient volume reaches beyond office or clinic capacity, costs rise even faster. This phenomenon is related to inefficiencies that occur in a sub-optimal environment (such as one with inadequate treatment space or redundant employees).

The above example is depicted in the "U" shaped cost curve on the following chart:

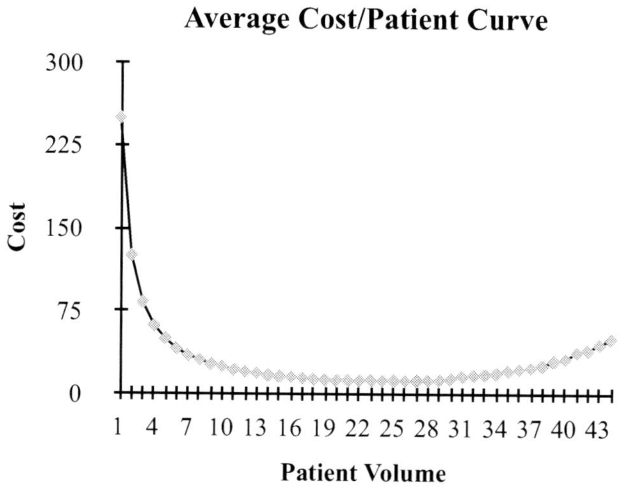

This curve is common to all businesses and shows clearly how the per patient cost initially drops quickly as patient volume increases and then tends to level off. An optimum point is reached when per patient costs level off to a minimum. This point is different for each practice and reflects over-all office efficiency. To determine this actual number for any particular practice, such factors as the number of treatment rooms, types of equipment available, business processes in place, treatment processes utilized, physician skills, and other factors that vary from clinic to clinic must be taken into account. This curve does not reflect revenue; however, no matter what the total revenue is at a given point in time, profit will be highest at the point on the cost curve where per patient costs are lowest.

Remember that the above graph represents *average* cost per patient. The reason that the speed of the decline of average cost slows, and then stops, is that at some point, the small incremental cost increase (marginal, or variable, cost) for new or additional business begins to "add up." This increase begins long before the average cost per patient begins to increase. The significant thing to understand here is that increasing patient volume beyond some optimal point has the actual potential of *reducing* the profit margin. There is some point at which more volume does not translate into more profit. The lower the fee, the sooner this point will be reached.

Fixed Costs and Variable Costs

It is essential to understand that there are two types of costs relevant to making decisions regarding volume or pricing: fixed and variable ones. Most data we receive from our accountants gives us only average and total costs. Both average and total cost numbers combine fixed and variable costs together. For most of the decisions we will be making – such as short-term pricing and contracting decisions that will alter patient volume – the variable costs are the ones that are relevant. Variable costs are the existing ones that will change as a direct result of implementing specific decisions.

Fixed costs, on the other hand, are the ones that are not going to be altered by a specific decision. They are a result of previous decisions and are the costs that are not going to change as a result of this new decision. Fixed costs should not be a factor when determining what changes you want to make. Using fixed costs when making short-term, strategic financial decisions leads to poor financial choices, especially when the choice involves whether or not to accept a contract that will increase patient volume.

For example: a doctor with a practice grossing $200,000 a year considers signing a contract that will increase the practice by 2,000 visits a year. The contract will add revenue of $25 per patient and, therefore, should increase revenue by $50,000. Before accepting the contract, the doctor needs to determine the cost of treating these additional patients.

The doctor's accountant analyzes the contract and recommends that it be rejected because, as he tells the doctor, "You will lose money." He explains that the practice overhead ($120,000) is 60 percent of total revenues and that the doctor had 4,000 patient visits last year (80 a week). From these figures, he calculates the average cost per patient to be $30 and informs the doctor that with the new contract's revenue of only $25 a patient, s/he would be losing $5 a patient.

While there may be other reasons for rejecting this contract, lack of profitability should not be one of them. Otherwise intelligent people often make this type of mistake. Fixed costs have not been correctly accounted for in making this decision.

Assume that the doctor will be able to accommodate the additional 2,000 patient visits (8 a day) without adding costs for more space or hiring additional employees. Further, assume that there is an average $3 supply cost for each patient ($6,000 for 2,000 patients). For purposes of this contract decision, rent, salaries, malpractice premiums, automobile expenses, telephone costs, and other expenses should not change. In other words, for purposes of this decision, these are all fixed expenses that should not enter into the decision making process because they will need to be paid whether or not the doctor accepts the contract. By considering only relevant costs (the variable ones, i.e. supply costs), the doctor determines that this contract will not produce a loss. Instead, it should increase profit by $44,000. This is demonstrated in *Table 1.1*.

Table 1.1: Calculating Contract Profitability

	Revenue	Overhead	Profit	% Profit Increase
Without Contract	$200,000	$120,000	$80,000	
Changes Under Contract	+ $50,000	+ $6,000	+ $44,000	
With Contract	**$250,000**	**$126,000**	**$124,000**	**55%**

If the doctor determines that treating these additional patients will require hiring one more employee, that employee's salary becomes a variable cost and is relevant to making the decision as to whether or not s/he should accept the contract. (The amount of this new salary would be added to the *overhead/changes under contract* entry in *Table 1.1*).

Confusion is created when some costs that we traditionally see as "fixed" become "variable" because of a particular change we are considering. For example, when making a decision regarding change in a practice, rent is usually considered a fixed expense; however, if a contract or merger is being considered which will increase patient volume to the point that the practice will require additional space, any resultant increase in rent is relevant to the decision being made. The amount of the rent *increase* is added to the variable costs at this point. If the current rent is $3,000 a month and the new rent would be $4,500 a month, the original $3,000 cost remains as a fixed expense while the $1,500 increase becomes a variable expense for purposes of this decision.

Revisiting the Profit Equation

Recall the profit equation: Profit = (Price ∗ Volume) - Cost. From what we now know about costs, we could re-write this equation as follows:

Profit = (Price ∗ Volume) - (Fixed Costs + Variable Costs)

This is the equation for total profit, but most decisions regarding fees and volume are based on predicted marginal (additional) profit. For these decisions, fixed costs are irrelevant and should not be included in the equation. The profit equation can be re-written as follows:

Marginal Profit = (Price x Increase in Volume) - Variable Costs

It is important to re-emphasize that the relevant costs for decision making vary with the type of decision being made. In the above contract and volume example, variable costs are the relevant ones. Later, we will see that fixed-costs are relevant when we are making cost cutting and efficiency improvement decisions.

Marginal Profit and Diminishing Returns

Assume that a clinic spends $20,000 for advertising in one year and that this advertising brings in 100 new patients, at an average of $300 per patient. This generates total additional revenue of $30,000. This $20,000 expenditure produces a net gain (profit) of $10,000. The average advertising cost, per new patient acquired, is $200, and the average revenue, per new patient, is $300.

Table 1.2: Marginal Profit from Advertising Cost

Advertising Cost	New Patients	Revenue Per Patient	Total New Revenue	Profit
$20,000	100	$300	$30,000	$10,000

Should the clinic have additional slack time in which to see more patients, it might make the strategic decision to increase next year's advertising by another $10,000. Using the available accounting data, this would seem to make sense; however, the clinic does not have all cost data necessary for making this decision. For example, what if, in the previous year, the first $10,000 spent had brought in 80 of the new patients? This would mean that the second $10,000 brought in only 20! Before making any decision, this practice needs to do a cost effectiveness analysis of its advertising expenditure.

This example alerts us to the fact that we should take into account the law of diminishing marginal returns: when making any financial decision, each additional dollar we spend beyond an optimum point has a decreasing return. In this case, the first $10,000 spent on advertising brought in $24,000 in revenue whereas the second $10,000 brought in only $6,000. With a loss of $4,000 for the second $10,000, it is clear that spending this second $10,000 was not cost-effective. This conclusion would not be clear if we were to use only total cost and average cost data.

Using the typical accounting data available to managers, this clinic would make the decision to spend an additional $10,000 on advertising – with the expectation of receiving 50 more new patients and $15,000 more in revenue; however, using the relevant numbers (incremental or marginal numbers), an optimal financial decision will be made: spend $10,000 less on advertising than last year. In this case, this year's advertising costs would be $10,000, and the benefit could be predicted to be $24,000 (80 * $300). This decision should result in $14,000 in profit – more than the previous year's $10,000.

Table 1.3: Comparison of Marginal Profit

New Patients	Revenue Per Patient	Total Revenue	Profit
100	$300	$30,000	$10,000
80	$300	$24,000	$14,000

Compare this with a decision to increase the $20,000 advertising budget by another $10,000 for the next year (a decision that is likely to be made when using only average and total cost data). This would bring the yearly advertising costs to $30,000, with a possible benefit of $33,000 (110 * 300). This produces a profit of only $3,000 as compared to the potential $14,000 in profit to be achieved by *reducing* the budget by $10,000 in the next year!

Table 1.4: Returns on Diverse Advertising Costs

Advertising Cost	New Patients	Revenue Per Patient	Total Revenue	Profit
$30,000	120	$300	$33,000	$3,000
$20,000	100	$300	$30,000	$10,000
$10,000	80	$300	$24,000	$14,000

Opportunity Costs

When making decisions, there are implied costs to consider that do not appear on financial statements. Every time we make a decision, we are choosing between alternatives, and there are always tradeoffs when choosing one alternative over another. For example, when we choose to schedule a procedure from 8:30 to 10:30, we exclude other types of patient care between those hours. Or, if we add space to our business office, we exclude the possibility of using that same space for patient treatment. Making a decision requires tradeoffs. One measure of the cost of a decision is the amount of profit that might be lost as a result of that decision – profit that would have been earned had an alternative choice been made. This cost is referred to as *opportunity cost*, and it can be incurred even when no money is spent. Opportunity cost will not show up on a profit/loss statement, but it should be considered when making a decision regarding the use of time, capital, or space.

If someone in a practice is performing one function, it is always at the exclusion of other possible choices. For example, if a back office assistant is drawing blood, he or she cannot be changing a dressing or taking an x-ray at the same time. A dollar amount can always be put on "the best alternative foregone," and obviously, one's time should always be spent on the highest valued opportunity (in some cases, using a doctor's free time may even be the most valued opportunity). Sometimes, choices involving opportunity costs are made "on the spot," and at others, they are the result of extensive analysis and planning. Opportunity costs become most relevant when re-engineering a practice because many of the decisions made during the re-engineering process involve "who does what and when."

In the early seventies, "The $100,000 Practice" was a goal to be achieved. I recall a well-known practice management expert stating, " If your practice is generating $100,000 a year, your time is worth $50 an hour. A $50 per hour doctor should not be doing $10 an hour work." This statement might "sound right" on cursory hearing, but it does not take opportunity costs into account, and adhering rigidly to such advice can result in creating support staffs (who do the "less than $50 per hour" work) that are too large, costly, and less efficient than ones that are smaller and better-trained.

There is always potential for making a wrong decision when basing that decision on *averages*. For example, in the course of a typical day there may be a few hours when a doctor who averages $50 an hour is actually producing $400 an hour and other times when s/he is producing nothing. At the times when there are no opportunities to produce income, the doctor's opportunity costs are zero. At such times, we do not want that doctor to interrupt an assistant who is already performing productive work in order to ask him or her to perform a task (a less than $50 per hour one) which the idled doctor could easily perform (i.e. remove a dressing or even schedule a return appointment from a computer terminal located in the treatment room). If such a need occurs at a time when the doctor's opportunity costs are zero, it is the doctor who is the best person to perform that task at that moment. While some of these tasks may seem to be relatively "insignificant," failure to consider the doctor's opportunity costs in such "small matters" can result in substantial cost increases in a practice and overall inefficiencies. A "micropractice" consisting of one doctor, one nurse, and maximum use of information technology is an extreme example of allocating physician and staff time based primarily on opportunity costs.

Sunk Costs

Sunk costs are the final ones to consider when making strategic decisions. They are different from fixed costs in that they are those costs that will not be changed as a result of making a strategic decision (even over the long-term). For this reason, sunk costs should never be a factor when making such a decision. For example, assume that you purchase a computer system at a cost of $32,000. Four years later, that system needs to be upgraded – at a cost of $16,000. A brand new system, which has the same capabilities as can be obtained through upgrading this old system, can be purchased for $9,000. Should the doctor purchase the new system and scrap the old one – or should he upgrade the old system?

I have seen some very intelligent people choose to upgrade old systems at a time like this, arguing that they do not want to lose the money they have already invested. In this case, the $32,000 is a *sunk cost* and should be considered irrelevant to making the decision. Assuming that the upgrade is essential to the practice, the relevant decision is whether it would be better to spend $9,000 (the new system) or $16,000 (the upgrade) to achieve a fully functional computer system that is capable of meeting the practice's current demands.

Initially, the answer to the above problem might seem obvious; however, this type of problem can assume many forms, and doctors frequently make poor financial decisions when such a choice arises. Assume that the money for the $32,000 computer system had been borrowed, employing a ten-year bank note at an annual interest rate of 9%. The payments are $405.36 a month, and there are six years remaining on the loan payments. Over the next six years the doctor will pay out $29,185.92 ($405.36 * 12 * 6 = $29,185.92). Does this change the decision being made? Initially, it might seem like a game changer, and yet, the loan and the monthly payments are actually irrelevant to the decision and should not be considered when making it. The loan is a sunk cost; it must be paid, regardless of which decision is made (this loan repayment is common to both decisions). The loan payments are relevant for cash flow planning but not for this strategic financial decision.

A final comment on sunk costs: when sunk costs are involved, emotion often enters the picture and confuses the decision-making process. If someone has invested a great deal of time or money – usually both – in an idea or a product, it is difficult to "let go" of that idea or product. This is why it can be difficult to sell a losing stock and replace it with a winner. There is plenty of room in clinical medicine for emotion, but there is no place for emotion when making strategic financial decisions.

Andy Grove, former CEO of Intel, has put forth the interesting strategy of "firing yourself" to remove the emotional component of sunk costs in his 1996 book, *Only the Paranoid Survive*. He tells the story of a time when Intel was losing market share of its memory chip business to Asian competitors. At the time, memory chips were the foundation of Intel's business, and the company was setting out to "beat the competition at their own game"; they were going to make a better chip and sell it for less. It soon became clear that this strategy was not working and that it probably never would. Grove realized that he and his management team carried too much baggage to think this situation through logically and unemotionally and asked his colleague, Gordon Moore, "If we got kicked out and the board brought in a new CEO, what do you think he would do?" Moore's answer, "He would get us out of the memory chip business." Grove responded by asking, "Why shouldn't you and I walk out the door, come back and do that ourselves?" This is precisely what they did, and Intel soon began focusing on the production of microprocessors, which reignited the company's growth and led to even greater success. Since the publication of Grove's book, many CEOs have adopted this approach.

While "firing and re-hiring yourself" may sound simple, this way of thinking offers a powerful approach to strategic planning. In most companies, new CEOs and management teams come in and make the changes that the previous CEO and management already knew needed to be made. A wise sage once said, "It is hard to see the writing on the wall when your back is up against it." "Firing yourself" frees you from past baggage and forces you to turn around and read that writing on the wall. Once you see what needs to be done, appropriate strategies will soon follow.

Determining Relevant Costs

To gain a better understanding of which costs should be used when making financial decisions, let us examine some everyday examples outside of medicine. A simple example is the situation that arises when an out-of-town relative is coming to stay in your guest room for a week. If your house payments are $30,000 a year ($577 a week), utilities are $300 a month ($75 a week), food is $420 a week, and extra food for the guest will cost $30 a day ($210 a week), what will this guest's one week's stay cost you?

Table 1.5: Weekly Housing Expense

	House Payment	Utilities	Food	Opportunity Cost	Weekly Guest Cost
Fixed Cost	$577	$75	$420	$0	$0
Variable Cost	$0	$0	$210	$0	$210

From this data, an accountant might calculate a cost for one week at $862.

Accountant's Math:

$557 + $75 + $210 = $862

However, we intuitively know that it doesn't really cost us this much. In this decision, the rent and utility costs are fixed and should be irrelevant to making the decision. The only relevant cost in this decision is the variable one of $210 for food.

What if you normally rent the guest room for $577 a week? This changes the decision being made. The guest room is no longer a fixed cost. Having a relative stay in the guest room now costs you the lost opportunity of earning $577 in rent. This is the *opportunity cost* of having your relative stay, and this lost opportunity is easily quantifiable. In this example, the cost of having the guest increases from $210 to $787 ($210 + $577).

Table 1.6: Guest Room Opportunity Cost

	House Payment	Utilities	Food	Opportunity Cost	Weekly Guest Cost
Fixed Cost	$577	$75	$420	$0	$0
Variable Cost	$0	$0	$210	$577	$787

Let us consider a second example. An airline has a flight from Los Angeles to New York at a price of $400 per passenger. There are 300 seats available on the plane, and 296 are filled. For this flight, the costs are as follows: pilot and nine support personnel, $6,000;

gasoline, $15,000; food, $4,440 ($15 per passenger); ground crew, $5,000; and one day's payment on the plane's loan, $12,000. The total cost of the flight is $42,440 ($143.38 per passenger). Four passengers arrive at the last minute and are willing to pay $100 each for the flight.

Table 1.7: Airline Cost/Seat

Cost	Pilot & Crew	Gas	Food	Ground Crew	Plane Loan	Cost per Seat
Fixed	$6,000	$15,000	$4,440	$5,000	$12,000	$143.38
Variable	$0.00	$0.00	$60.00	$0.00	$0.00	$15.00

If the airline discounts the rate from $400 to $100 for these four passengers, will it lose or make money? The airline's accountant argues that they will lose $173.52 by discounting the rate for the four passengers.

Accountant's Figures:

Revenue = $100.00 ∗ 4 = $400.00
Cost = $143.38 ∗ 4 = $573.52
Profit = $400.00 - $573.52 = ($173.52)

For this decision, however, every cost, other than the additional meals, is fixed. If the food for 300 passengers is already on the plane, even the cost of food is fixed. If the airline needs to add four meals, the only cost of adding four more passengers is the variable $60 cost of those meals (4 ∗ $15= $60). The opportunity cost is zero because, at this moment, there is no alternative opportunity to sell the seats for more money. The fixed costs are irrelevant to this decision. The $12,000 loan payment is not only a fixed cost, it is a sunk one. If the food is already on the plane, the airline will make an additional profit of $400 by discounting the remaining four seats, rather than losing $173.52 on the deal as some might assume. Failing to fill the last four seats at a discounted price of $100 each is a $400 profit-opportunity lost to the airline.

We intuitively know that a plane about to take off with four empty seats will not lose money by selling the remaining seats at a discount. This "discount at the margin" is profitable, and if, in this case, the food is already on the plane, increasing the number of passengers from 296 to 300 will cost the airline nothing.

Consider a second scenario: what if five passengers, instead of four, show up at the last minute wanting a discount? Increasing the number of passengers from 300 to 301 creates an entirely different situation. To fly one more passenger beyond the 300 requires commissioning another plane and adding nine more crew. The airline will not add another flight unless it can cover all costs. The decision now becomes, "How many additional passengers are needed, and what should the airline charge each passenger, in order to add one more flight and have it be profitable?" In making this decision, almost all the costs that were fixed in the previous example become variable.

Table 1.8: Airline Break-Even Cost per Seat

Cost	Pilot & Crew	Gas	Food	Ground Crew	Plane Loan	Cost Per Seat
Fixed	$0.00	$0.00	$0.00	$5,000	$12,000	
Variable	$6,000	$15,000	$4,440	$0.00	$0.00	$84.80

The total accounting cost calculated previously for adding this flight is $42,440. However, the $12,000 plane loan portion of this total is a "sunk cost" and is not relevant to making the decision. The airline will have more incentive to add the flight if there will be some contribution of money to the fixed and sunk costs. If it is able to use the same ground crew, that $5,000 cost is fixed. The relevant total cost that the airline must cover to make a profit is $25,440 (the sum of all the variable costs in the chart above), and if the airline were to fill all 300 seats, the break-even ticket cost would be $84.80 per seat (*Table 1.8*).

The airline faces a pricing dilemma. If it cannot cover the minimum variable costs of $25,440 (pilot, crew, gas, and food) it must cancel the flight. It would like to cover the full cost of $42,440 (which includes the ground crew and plane loan) – plus make a profit; however, it would not make sense financially for the airline to cancel the flight if revenue between $25,440 and $42,440 could be generated because any revenue within this range would contribute toward fixed costs (marginal profit for the airline). The airline would like to set an initial ticket price that would cover all costs and produce a desired amount of profit. The higher the ticket price, the lower the demand will be. If the flight is full, a price of $141.47, or more, per seat will cover all variable and fixed costs. The airline must now use market data to decide what price above $141.47 will produce the most profit. For example, will they be able to fill the plane at $200 per seat, or will a flight that is three-quarters full, at $300 per seat, be more profitable? Once the flight is profitable, the airline can increase its profit by discounting the remaining seats.

Consider a final scenario: what if the airline discounts all 300 seats to $80? Rather than discounting at the margin, this is a "discount to the core." Discounting on the margin is always profitable. Discounting to the core would result in total revenue of $24,000 (300 * $80). We previously calculated that the total cost of this flight is $42,440. $12,000 of this cost is a "sunk" loan payment, and the $5,000 ground crew cost is fixed. In this case, the airline should consider canceling the flight because, with total revenue of $24,000, and variable costs of $25,440, this flight would lose the airline $1,440. If the variable cost of providing a service cannot be recovered in revenue, the additional business should be declined. Pricing below variable costs is referred to as "predatory pricing," and large companies occasionally use this tactic to gain market share or to drive competitors out of business. In a medical practice, this would be comparable to paying a vendor $150 for a DME product and then dispensing it to a patient for $130. In this example the correct decision is obvious because the marginal cost is obvious. In decisions involving volume and pricing changes, marginal cost is not as obvious, but it will still have the same impact on profit.

Tying It All Together: Using Relevant Costs to Make Decisions in Your Practice

Let us relate the above airline example to a medical facility that is considering a discounted contract. All discount contract decisions are similar to the example above. The key question to ask is, "Does this contract call for a discount at the margin or a discount to the core?" It is essential that you make this determination because the relevant costs will be different depending on the type of discount you will be dealing with.

When analyzing potential contracts, think of your office as an airplane with some empty seats. These empty seats represent unfilled treatment rooms and openings in your patient schedule. If the contract being considered is a discount at the margin, it is intended to supply you with additional patients who will "fill the empty seats." Your costs for rent, staff, malpractice insurance, equipment, and most other expenses are irrelevant for making this decision because they are fixed. The only cost that you need to consider when estimating whether or not the contract will be profitable is the variable expense of the additional medical supplies needed to treat the new patients the contract will bring in.

If the contract supplies your practice with an increase in patient flow so large that you require more staff, an additional doctor, or a physician extender, their new salary expenses are considered variable and become relevant for purposes of estimating profit. They will be added to the cost for supplies needed for the new patients. All other expenses are fixed and are not relevant to the decision. If the contract is so large that, when in place, it would provide the majority of your practice's patients, all costs become variable for purposes of the decision and must be covered by the contract. You would use the same approach when considering a merger of two or more practices "under the same roof." This is not an exact science; however, if you understand these airline examples, you will be able to make significantly better financial decisions.

If you begin breaking down financial cost decisions into categories which include: opportunity, fixed, variable, and sunk costs, you will be well on your way to developing an "economic mind set" rather than an "emotional mind set." Even at this point, if you thoroughly understand the material already presented, you should have a better understanding for making cost decisions than many CPAs.

Chapter 2

Use Leverage to Your Advantage

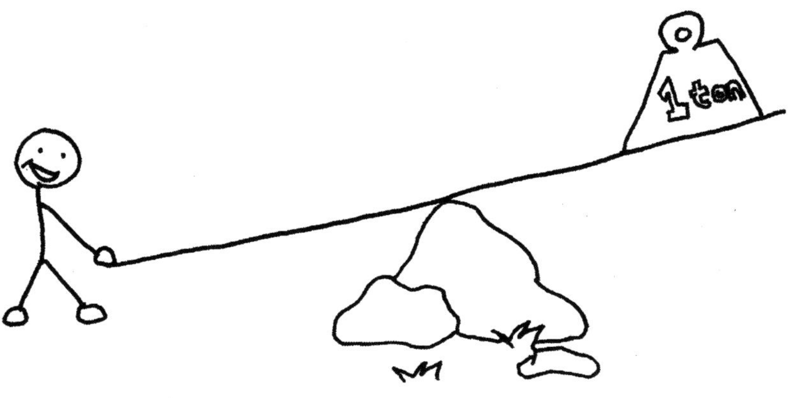

Leverage for Non-Physicists

We all are aware of *leverage* from our studies in physics – a mechanical advantage gained through use of a tool. For example, a lever allows us to move a heavy object by applying a relatively small amount of force. We can also apply this term to a medical practice in which case a gain in finances or treatment quality might be magnified as a result of using a superior process or "strategy." Utilization of a superior process leverages any practice's revenue gains – creating disproportionate gains in profit. When the revenue of a well-run medical practice grows, the percentage increase in profit should always outpace the percentage increase in revenue. This effect of magnifying profit is the result of "operating leverage," with the caveat being that leverage will magnify the impact of any change in revenue – including one in a negative direction.

In order to succeed in an environment in which prices are declining and costs are increasing, it is important for a doctor to have an understanding of this power of leverage. Here is a familiar example of the term leverage as it applies to finances – in this case, the purchase of a home. Assume that we purchase a $1,000,000 home, investing $100,000 (10%) as a down payment. Our $100,000 investment is leveraged as the home price increases. When the home's value reaches $1,100,000 (a 10% increase), our $100,000 investment has grown 100% – increasing from $100,000 to $200,000. In this case, our investment has provided us with a financial leverage of ten to one. Financial leverage can also have a downside. If, conversely, the value of this $1,000,000 home were to sink to $900,000 (a 10% decrease), 100% of our original investment would be lost. With the advantage of understanding the potential advantages and disadvantages of leverage, let us look at how it can work to our benefit in a medical practice.

A Quick Word of Caution on Percentages

In spite of the fact that a pre-med education includes a significant number of courses in math and science, physicians often struggle with numbers when they are followed by a percent sign. In many cases, we simply do not take sufficient time to fully appreciate the context in which a percentage is being used, and this can lead to misinterpretation. Since we often deal with percentages, let's take the time to see common areas where we might err in their use. I have selected two examples to demonstrate how misinterpretation is possible when we do not take the time to question how a percentage is being used in a specific situation.

Percent Change versus Percentage Point Change

A useful strategy for increasing a medical practice's revenue is to work on increasing its collection percentage. A significant issue here is that many doctors confuse "percentage increase" with "percentage point increase," creating a situation in which apples might mistakenly be compared to oranges. For example, assume a practice with annual gross charges of $800,000 and a collection percentage of 38%. The resultant revenue is $304,000 (38% * $800,000 = $304,000). A consultant examines the practice's collection process and estimates that by streamlining this process, its ratio can be increased 12%. What would the new collection ratio and the new revenue be if the doctor were able to accomplish this feat? S/he might assume this percentage increase to mean that the collection ratio would simply increase to 50% (38% + 12%). In reality, it would increase from 38.00% to 42.56% [38% + (38% * 12%) = 42.56%], and the revenue collected would increase from $304,000 to $340,480 ($800 * 42.56% = $340,480), not $400,000 ($800,000 * 50% = $400,000) – as some might expect. In fact, growing revenue from $304,000 to $400,000 would require an increase of *12 percentage point*s in the collection ratio rather than a 12% increase. This greater amount of $96,000 ($400,000 - $304,000) would be obtained if the collection ratio were 50%, and this would require a 31.58% increase in the starting ratio of 38.00% [38% + (31.58% * 38%) = 50%] – much greater than the consultant had estimated as "doable."

With Percentages, Increases are not Equivalent to Decreases

It is easy to overlook the fact that percentages do not directly translate when comparing ones defining increases to ones quantifying decreases. For example, assume that the stock market suddenly drops 20% and then turns around – increasing 20%, the following week. Have you recovered all of your losses? The answer is "no"; yet, not everyone finds this intuitive.

Let us examine this question by starting with the example of a $100,000 portfolio. Assume, as above, that the market drops 20%. Our portfolio's value is now $80,000. If the $80,000 in this portfolio were then to turn around and grow 20%, the value would increase to $96,000. Note that we are not at our starting point of $100,000. In order to recover our full 20% loss of $20,000, the market would actually have to increase 25% from its low point (25% * $80,000 = $20,000).

How might this concept apply to our practices? We must recognize that drops in medical fees impact our practice revenues in this same manner. If all our fees were cut by 20%, we would need to increase total charges by 25% (not 20%) in order to recover the income loss created by the fee decrease and be back where we started.

Those who have lost significant portions of their retirement plans due to stock market declines have been through a "real world" experience demonstrating this same dynamic. As an example, between January 1, 2008, and March 9, 2009, the market dropped 50.64%, and from March 10 through June 10, 2009, it increased 33.48%. While this was a nice increase, its end results were not as great as some assumed. If we were again to use our $100,000 portfolio as the example and drop its value by this 50.64%, its new value would be $49,360. While some might think that the market would "only" have to increase 50.64%, in order to recover the full 50.64% decline that had occurred, we now realize that the market would actually have to increase 102.61% from its low point. This is what it would take to return our portfolio back to its January 2008 starting point of $100,000 [$49,360 + ($49,360 * 102.61%) = $100,000]. Misinterpretations are easily made in any situation such as this where percentages representing increases are compared to ones representing decreases. Be careful not to make similar misinterpretations when comparing percentage changes in your practice (such as changes in patient volume, revenue, or overhead); keep in mind that the uphill climb is greater than the downhill fall.

The Leverage of Increasing Fees

A fee increase provides a medical practice with leverage for increasing profitability. Consider a sample practice with $400,000 in revenue, $240,000 in expenses, and $160,000 in profit (*Table 2.1*). If this practice were able to increase its fees by 20%, while keeping costs the same, revenue would increase the expected 20% (from $400,000 to $480,000); however, profit would increase from $160,000, to $240,000 – a 50% increase!

Table 2.1: Increasing Fees 20%

	Before Increase	After 20% Increase	Percent Change
Revenue	$400,000	$480,000	20.00%
Expenses	$240,000	$240,000	0.00%
Profit	$160,000	$240,000	50.00%

Conversely, a fee decrease provides leverage in the opposite direction – negatively! If fees were decreased 20% for this practice, revenue would drop 20% (from $400,000 to $320,000), and profit would decrease from $160,000, to $80,000 – a 50% decrease (*Table 2.2*)!

Table 2.2: Decreasing Fees 20%

	Before Decrease	After 20% Decrease	Percent Change
Revenue	$400,000	$320,000	-20.00%
Expenses	$240,000	$240,000	0.00%
Profit	$160,000	$80,000	-50.00%

Although fees seem to move only in a downward direction, it is important to note that at any given time, the amount paid for the same service varies from doctor to doctor. In general, IPAs have been able to negotiate better rates than individual doctors, and large group practices often receive the top rates. Given a future in which many services will be non-covered, patients will be required to pay cash, and the amount paid by insurance companies for covered services will be based on documented quality, rather than quantity, it behooves a doctor to factor in the advantages of leverage when determining where to spend his/her time and effort when preparing for the future.

The Leverage of Improving Collection Efficiencies

Medical practices are generally high-fixed-cost businesses. Fortunately, the variable costs are low. In a model such as this, either raising prices and/or increasing volume offers us leverage in our attempts to increase profit. While raising fees is not an option in the price-competitive medical market (except for non-covered services or concierge and "cash only" type practices), such "tactics" as coding correctly, capturing all billable charges, collecting cash for non-covered services at the time of visits, avoiding errors, developing an optimum payer and service mix – all things which either increase productivity and/or the collection ratio – provide a practice with financial leverage similar to that achieved by raising fees. For example, a practice that has a 60% overhead and makes improvements in 20% of these areas will experience a leveraged impact on profit of 50% without increasing patient volume. *Table 2.3* shows the before-and-after picture of a practice with a 60% overhead that, through successful implementation of efficiencies, a 10% increase in its capture of charges, and a 9.1% increase in its collection ratio, realizes a 50% profit improvement (from $167,000 to $250,466).

Table 2.3: Increase in Charge Capture & Collection Ratio

	Before	After	% Change
Charge Capture	$1,097,368	$1,207,105	10.0%
Collection %	38.00%	41.46%	9.1%
Collections	$417,000	$500,466	20.0%
Overhead	$250,000	$250,000	0.0%
Profit	$167,000	$250,466	50.0%
Overhead Ratio	60.0%	50.0%	(16.7%)

This practice has successfully increased its profit by increasing collections while keeping its costs stable. Most busy practices have significant inefficiencies in their billing processes that, if improved, could easily add 20% to their collections. Since improved efficiency in this area does not require an increase in volume, there is no change in fixed or variable costs, creating significant leverage for increasing profit.

The Leverage of Increasing Patient Volume

To demonstrate the leverage that an increase in volume can have on a high, fixed-cost business such as medicine, consider a practice with the following statistics: 1) a fixed overhead of $250,000, 2) an average, per patient, variable cost of $6, and 3) an average, per patient, revenue of $100. If this practice were to see just one patient over an entire year, the average, per patient, cost would be $250,006 (the $250,000 fixed cost plus the variable cost of $6 for each patient), and the average, per patient, revenue would be $100. In this example, $250,006 would also be the total annual cost, and $100 would be the total revenue. If two patients were seen, the cost, per patient, would drop almost 50% – from $250,006 to $125,006 ($250,012 ÷ 2 = $125,006), while total costs would increase minimally – from $250,006 to $250,012. Annual revenue would double, from $100 to $200. As volume increases, this leverage continues – even though total costs increase. This is because the total costs increase slowly while the average cost, per patient, decreases rapidly.

A practice's "bottom line" financial figure – its goal – is profit. In order for our example practice to break-even and move towards profitability, it must reach an annual volume of 2,660 patient visits (see *Table 2.4*). Each visit beyond this break-even point adds $100 in revenue while increasing expenses by only $6. The resultant marginal profit rate is $94 per visit. From the break-even point forward, we can see the impact that each incremental volume increase of 10% will have on profit. The chart below shows us the tremendous profit leverage that increased volume offers in these early stages of building a practice. Even at the level where volume is almost double that of the break-even point, there is profit leverage of more than two to one.

Table 2.4: Leverage Past Break-Even

Patient Volume	Total Cost	Total Revenue	Total Profit	% Profit Increase
2,660	**$265,957**	**$265,957**	**$0**	**(break-even)**
2,926	$267,553	$292,553	$25,000	-
3,218	$269,308	$321,808	$52,500	110%
3,540	$271,240	$354,000	$82,760	58%
3,894	$273,364	$389,400	$116,036	40%
4,283	$275,698	$428,300	$152,602	32%
4,711	$278,266	$471,100	$192,834	26%
5,182	$281,092	$518,200	$237,108	23%

If a practice continues to grow, it will eventually reach a volume level at which either additional staff or office space must be added – either of which will increase fixed costs and thereby, initially, decrease profit. This point will occur at much higher patient volume levels for practices that have implemented efficient processes because improving the efficiency of business processes will assist a practice in maintaining its existing fixed costs at higher volume levels. Improved efficiency will also increase the percentage of charges captured as well as the collection ratio, both of which have the same leveraged impact on profit as does an increase in volume. Given that most practices charge more than twice what they expect to collect, a collection ratio of 40% needs to be increased only a few percentage points to achieve the same leverage as a 10% increase in volume.

What strategy makes the most sense in a price competitive environment? There is no question that an increase in volume, combined with improvements in efficiency, provides a practice with the greatest amount of leverage for increasing profit. Given a future environment of increased demand, coupled with declining numbers of physicians, practices are likely to grow in volume each year. This increase, coupled with improved efficiency, should provide substantial profit leverage. A strategy that provides dramatic leverage almost "overnight" (utilizing both increased volume and improved efficiency) is a simple merger of practices. This not only provides the leverage of an immediate volume increase but also an opportunity to quickly reduce fixed costs (since costs such as rent and per doctor staffing ratios should reduce following a merger). Regardless of what your current level of patient volume and profitability may be, when planning goals and strategies for the future, it will be motivating to determine the impact that a 10% volume increase, combined with a 4% increase in the collection ratio, would have on your profitability.

The Leverage of Reducing Cost Versus that of Increasing Revenue

Cost cutting will provide more leverage for increasing profit than increasing revenue, especially in an environment of discounted fees. The leverage provided by cost cutting is especially great in practices that have steadily grown in volume without addressing inefficiencies, thereby allowing an accumulation of unnecessary costs to occur. Consider a practice that has $1,000,000 in total revenue and $666,700 in total costs (a 66.67% overhead). A 10% cost reduction would result in $66,670 additional profit (0.10 * $666,700 = $66,670) – a 20% profit increase. Assuming a constant overhead of 66.67%, a 20% revenue increase ($200,000) would be another way to achieve this same profit increase of $66,670 (.6667 * $200,000 = $133,340 and $200,000 - $133,330 = $66,660). The profit is the same using either strategy, but achieving a revenue increase by increasing volume necessitates that the doctor manage a substantial number of additional patients.

Table 2.5: 2:1 Cost Reduction Leverage

Practice Change	Revenue	Costs	Profit	% Profit Change
Original	$1,000,000	$666,700	$333,300	-
10% Cost ↓	$1,000,000	$600,030	$399,970	+20%
20% Revenue ↑	$1,200,000	$800,040	$399,960	+20%

In this constant overhead ratio example, either a 10% reduction in costs or a 20% increase in revenue will produce the same increase in profit. With a 33% gross profit margin, cost reduction provides a leverage of 2 to 1 over a revenue increase!

You can apply this principle when considering opting into or out of a contract. It is possible to have a variety of contracts all paying different rates. As any contracted rate lowers, its contribution to profit (marginal profit) decreases. When faced with the decision of whether to opt into, or out of, a contract, it is helpful to compare that contract's projected contribution to profit with the lowest percentage cost-reduction needed to provide an equal amount of profit. Again, the smaller the contract's profit margin the greater the leverage you have through cost-reduction.

Consider the practice in the above example with the decision being whether to enter into a contract projected to increase total revenue by 20% ($200,000) at a cost of $160,000. The contract's projected profit contribution is $40,000 (a 20% profit margin), which will increase total profit by 12%. The cost reduction necessary to increase profit the same amount as this 20% revenue increase is only 6%. In this case, a 6% cost reduction produces results equivalent to a 20% revenue increase! With a profit margin of 20%, the leverage for cutting costs is now more than three to one over increasing revenue.

Table 2.6: Cost Reduction Leverage (Approximately 3:1)

Practice Change	Revenue	Costs	Profit	% Profit Change
Original	$1,000,000	$666,700	$333,300	-
6% Cost ↓	$1,000,000	$626,700	$373,300	+12%
20% Revenue ↑	$1,200,000	$826,700	$373,300	+12%

Profit margins for the same contract will vary from practice to practice, depending on the cost-position and efficiency level of each practice. There are some contracts being offered that may provide five percent profit margins for some practices, as shown in *Table 2.7*. In this case, a 1.5% cost reduction is equal to a revenue increase of 20%. With a profit margin of five percent, the leverage for cost cutting increases to thirteen to one.

Table 2.7: Cost Reduction Leverage (Approximately 13:1)

Practice Change	Revenue	Costs	Profit	% Profit Change
Original	$1,000,000	$666,700	$333,300	-
1.5% Cost ↓	$1,000,000	$656,700	$343,300	+3%
20% Revenue ↑	$1,200,000	$856,700	$343,300	+3%

These examples demonstrate that as a profit margin decreases, the leverage provided by cost cutting increases; yet, when practitioners are faced with declining incomes, most spend the majority of their time focusing on ways to increase volume and revenue rather than on ways to reduce costs. This is a carry-over from a time when medicine was in a growth market with high profit margins. In that type of market, it was correct for the doctor to focus primarily on revenue and secondarily on cost; however, this has changed.

Though today's market has changed, the majority of doctors continue to run their practices as they would have in the past. They focus on methods directed at producing more revenue although most are not suffering from lack of revenue, but rather, from lack of profit. Gross revenues are far higher than most doctors ever expected to generate when they first entered practice. Unfortunately, so are their overheads. In a mature, price competitive market such as we have today, a significant emphasis should be placed on increasing efficiency and eliminating unnecessary costs. The examples above demonstrate the leverage effects to be obtained from relatively modest cost reductions. Imagine the profit increase that a more radical cost reduction – say 20% to 30% – might achieve!

The Leverage of Spending Less

Typically, doctors obtain practice management insights from journal articles, lectures, newspapers, and conversations with peers. Occasionally, these insights "jump out" at us when least expected, such as in verses of songs or lines from movies. One example is a practice management insight that struck me when I saw the movie "Bandits." The film featured Billy Bob Thornton and Bruce Willis as two professional bank robbers. Following a lucrative bank heist, Thornton went on a spending spree, purchasing a host of luxury items that he didn't need. In order to "educate" him regarding the foolishness of his wasteful ways, Willis remarked: "Every dollar you spend is another dollar that we have to steal!" While this is a funny line in the context of the movie, it is one well stated. This line gives a fresh perspective and could serve as a guide for changing behavior and focus. Willis wants Thornton to focus on costs as well as on revenue. He recognizes the impact of each on the other. Doctors, too, could benefit from a focus on costs as well as revenue.

The fact that the relationship between revenue and costs is not a dollar for dollar one is a challenge for medical practitioners. If a movie were to be made that included a scene depicting two physician partners discussing the expenses of their medical practice, the Willis line would need to be changed to: "Every dollar you spend is another four dollars that we have to bill." Assume the following statistics for the average practice: 1) collection ratio = 77%, 2) overhead = 50%, and 3) tax rate = 35%. *Table 2.7* shows that only one dollar is available for personal spending for every four dollars billed. Unnecessary spending (overhead) must be controlled at the office, just as it must be at home. Regardless of where spending occurs, the end result is the same – four dollars must be billed to generate each dollar of take-home for the doctor. Each personal income dollar conserved is the same as billing four times the saved amount, and each $1.54 of overhead cost conserved produces the same result as billing an additional $4. This does not mean that a medical practice should discontinue marketing or stop increasing patient volume; however, given the upside leverage possible through controlling costs and reducing unnecessary expenses, these are strategies that should be given the greatest attention.

Table 2.7

Amount Billed	$4.00
Collect 77%	$3.08
After 50% Overhead	$1.54
After 35% Tax	$1.00

Table 2.8

Amount Billed	$8.00
Collect 48%	$3.84
After 65% Overhead	$1.34
After 35% Tax	$0.87

This four to one relationship for the average practice can become an eight to one relationship (especially in larger groups) if inefficiencies are not reduced. It is not unusual to see a larger group practice with a 65% overhead and a 48% collection ratio, resulting in less than one after-tax dollar for every eight billed (*Table 2.8*). Overhead is a necessary cost for providing medical services and producing revenue, but high overheads are typical and represent a significant burden for doctors. Controlling expenses does not require "being cheap" or putting off investing in a practice. It means selectively spending in areas that will increase quality and/or provide a return that is greater than the cost. Expenses that do not accomplish this end are wasteful, add no value, and should, therefore, be eliminated. Identifying these expenses and controlling them during periods of growth is healthy for a practice. This will provide greater profit leverage than that created by a much larger increase in revenue.

The Leverage of Spending More

There is a maxim in business often evoked when a company in financial trouble exclusively focuses on cost cutting as the solution. This maxim states, "You can't cut your way into prosperity." Spending money during a time that it is in short supply makes sense when there is an expected return, and should be considered as a part of any efficiency improvement strategy. Return on investment (ROI) is a relatively straightforward concept to understand as it applies to traditional financial investments, but it is more challenging to apply this concept to practice expenditure decisions where the source of potential return is ill defined. When we invest our hard-earned money in stocks, bonds, and savings accounts, we expect to make a financial return on our investments. Furthermore, we expect our financial return to be in proportion to the amount of risk we are taking; we expect a higher return from "risky" stocks than we do from "safe," insured savings accounts. Doctors would benefit significantly from viewing all practice expenditures as investments and evaluating the benefit of each potential expenditure, based on its level of risk and expected ROI.

Practice decisions such as whether to hire an associate or additional staff member, purchase software, upgrade hardware, add treatment rooms, purchase new equipment, advertise in various media, sell medical supplies to patients, or purchase shares in an ASC should all be approached in the same manner as any other investment – with a focus on the expected return. The return on this type of investment includes both financial and non-financial benefits, and both of these should be included in the evaluation when making decisions regarding any practice expenditure. Assets such as medical equipment and software lend themselves more easily to an "ROI approach" than those such as staff or treatment rooms; however, when a consistent framework is used to evaluate every expenditure, the odds are greatly increased that higher returns will be achieved and wasteful spending will be avoided. By using a formal, systematic approach every time you evaluate an expenditure for its potential ROI, you are "quantifying" each of your goals and setting the strategy for achieving it.

It happens too often that an expected financial return doesn't materialize. Doctors tend to rely on "sales pitches" (sometimes exaggerated) from equipment vendors rather than estimating potential ROI for themselves. In the case of expenditures whose returns are more difficult to quantify (such as hiring new staff or adding treatment space), doctors expect a return, but they have no clear understanding of how much to expect, where that return might come from, or what all the "returns" might include. They have unclear goals and an even less clear strategy of how to achieve them. This is where a more formal approach will help.

Before developing a framework for estimating the ROI for a proposed expenditure, a doctor must first understand the various sources of financial return from a medical practice expenditure. To produce a return, an expenditure must do one, or more, of the following: 1) increase the revenue billed, 2) increase the collection percentage, 3) free up physician and/or staff time, 4) expand office capacity, or 5) increase treatment or operational quality. Keeping these five basic areas of potential return in mind, a framework or "checklist" of all costs that can be utilized to estimate the expenditure's ROI can now be developed.

For example, if a doctor were considering the purchase of practice management software (fully integrated with an electronic medical record) and wanted to estimate its potential ROI, s/he would start by determining each area of the office workflow to which the software would be applied and then estimating how each application might impact any of the five areas listed above. For example, 1) total revenue billed might be increased by such things as creating potential for capturing all billable charges, providing correct coding and documentation, improving the service and payer mix, and seeing a higher volume of patients, 2) the collection ratio might be improved by such things as speeding up the billing cycle, collecting co-pays at check-in and patients' portions at check-out, and making fewer billing errors (each of which requires subsequent identification and re-work), 3) staffing ratios might be decreased by eliminating data entry and paper medical records and by reducing interruptions between staff members caused by their having insufficient information, 4) office capacity would be increased by such things as utilizing a computerized appointment book effectively, cross-training staff, and extending office hours, and 5) quality would be increased by such things as creating the ability to measure treatment outcomes, prevent errors, and track care – assuring that no patient follow-up would fall through the cracks.

To estimate the ROI for the purchase of software, every one of its features should be examined in this way. Each feature should be scrutinized to determine where it would be applied in the workflow and what it would specifically do to produce a return, and an attempt should be made to quantify that return as a specific dollar amount. ROI never comes from one big thing, but rather, from the summation of dozens of "small" things such as these, which add up to "one big thing."

A formal process – such as the one described above, which focuses on estimating ROI – should be applied to all new proposed practice expenditures greater than $1,000. These proposed expenditures might be for such things as 1) attending a workshop to learn a new skill, 2) buying a new piece of equipment, 3) enlarging office space, 4) investing in an ASC, or 5) hiring additional staff. A formal process will not only help a doctor make better decisions regarding potential practice expenditures, but it will help him/her identify expected goals and develop better strategies for implementing potential "purchases" to achieve those goals, assuring a greater chance that the desired ROI will be achieved upon implementation.

The Strategic Leverage of Economic Game Theory

Game Theory dates back to 1944 with the publishing of *Theory of Games and Economic Behavior* by mathematician John von Neumann and economist Oskar Morgenstern. Game Theory is a useful tool in business situations where the fortunes of players or companies are interdependent and decisions made by one will affect or influence decisions made by the others. This describes virtually every situation encountered in today's healthcare environment. Game Theory was brought to the forefront more recently in a 1995 article, "The Right Game: Use Game Theory to Shape Strategy," written by Adam Brandenburger (a Harvard Business School professor) and Barry Nalebuff (a Yale Business School professor). This article was followed by their 1996 book *Co-optition* which put forth the concept that a combination of cooperation and competition are inherent in most business situations.

Game Theory is demonstrated in the strategy used when playing competitive sports or games like chess and bridge. Using the type of strategic thinking necessary for game playing – combined with mathematic, economic, financial, statistic, operational and business management concepts – can lead to better business decisions for those employed in today's competitive healthcare environment. Game theory can provide significant leverage in a wide variety of strategic situations. Rapid changes in healthcare and technology require rapid, strategic responses, and this is where Game Theory excels. This type of thinking helps a "player" to understand what is going on and how to improve a situation strategically. Let's take a closer look at four Game Theory principles that I feel are indispensable tools, ones that can sharpen your thought process for making strategic decisions and simultaneously provide leverage.

Principle One: Look forward and reason backward

Yogi Berra has been attributed with the saying, "It's hard to make predictions, especially about the future." Business projections are typically made by analyzing historical data and then using a combination of subjective experience and objective tools taught in business schools (such as econometrics and regression analysis) to project forward. This approach is a useful exercise, but it rarely leads to a superior decision – especially when technology and the environment are changing as rapidly as they are for today's healthcare provider. Using historical data to project forward has been compared to having a blindfolded driver dependent on the eyes of a navigator looking out a car's rear window and telling the driver when to turn and what direction to go.

A Game Theory approach often contradicts conventional wisdom. In most games, the future is "forecast" by looking forward to a desired outcome, or goal, and then thinking backwards to determine the moves necessary to reach that goal. For example, a short-term goal in chess might be to remove a bishop that is positioned to interfere with the long-term goal of advancing towards the king. The thinking process is begun at the point where the bishop (the obstacle) is "gone," and from there, the player reasons backwards through the moves needed to reach this goal. Throughout the "backwards thinking" process, the player is forced to consider any moves the competitor might make to prevent the removal of the bishop at each step. In chess, moves are predicted, based on the assumption that the opponent is trying to win the game and is assessing your ability (strengths and weaknesses) in order to more accurately "predict" your moves. The same is true in business. We determine who the decision makers are and ascertain what we can about their motives and abilities. In business, we also add the assumption that a player "wins the game" by maximizing profit and that s/he makes moves based on reaching this goal.

While this approach may seem obvious, few people in the business world tend to think this way. Those who do so hold a significant advantage, and their decisions improve as they gain more experience and knowledge about their competitors.

Principle Two: Determine the value that you bring to the game

This one principle defines why the Physician Practice Management Industry (PPMCs) failed and why HMOs have not yet become the preferred healthcare model. Business is all about meeting the needs of customers and creating value in the process. Physicians perceived that the value they received from PPMCs was lower than the fees those companies charged them, and they do not feel that HMOs meet the customer service needs of patients. In fact, patients contend that customer service has only become worse. Most business situations require that a "player" have a good understanding of the value s/he brings to the other players. In other words, how does s/he meet the needs of customers and/or add to profit?

Business transactions require negotiations, and a critical first step in your negotiating process is determining the value that you bring to the table. In the "old days," some physicians took greater value from the "treatment game" (relative to other doctors) than they brought to it, simply by using higher paying treatment codes. In Game Theory, this strategy does not work – an operative principle of Game Theory is that players *cannot* take more value from a game than they bring to it. The importance of adopting this principle is that it clearly directs a player towards a strategy intended to make him/her a more valuable player.

The best way to determine the value a player brings to a game is to estimate the impact that would be made on the other players if s/he were removed from the game. Since the real game of business is about creating value, this can be an eye opener for a doctor – recognizing the true value (or lack of value) that he/she as a player actually brings to the "game." Undergoing this process will lead to a better strategy – one directed at finding ways of becoming a more valuable player.

Principle Three: Develop a perspective that focuses on the positions of the other players, rather than on your own

Unlike typical games where there are winners and losers, "business games" present an opportunity for developing strategies whereby everyone can win. This is the fun of "playing" these games. Finding moves that allow all payers to win can lead to positive outcomes, creating synergistic opportunities in which collaboration (such as strategic partnerships or sharing infrastructure) provides leverage that can benefit all companies involved – especially in areas that save cost or accelerate growth.

Game Theory changes the focus from egocentric (What's in this for me?) to allocentric (What's in this for us?). By placing yourself in the "minds" of the other players and assessing your value in terms of what you can bring to others, the game changes from win-lose (or even lose-lose) to win-win. This "strategy" has broad applications to all areas of healthcare delivery and will achieve its optimum results when all players – payers, doctors, and patients alike – win. By applying the principles of game theory, this optimum will be reached much sooner.

Principle Four: Can't win? Change the game

"Changing the game" is one of Game Theory's most powerful business strategy applications – especially when a player recognizes that the game s/he is playing is not one s/he can win. For me, changing the game is the backbone of business strategy and makes "getting there" more fun. This strategy can create opportunities that, at first, appear impossible.

It is important for players to recognize that when the deck is stacked against them, or other players are holding all the "good cards," they don't have to play the game they find themselves in. You may have faced such a situation – when applying for hospital privileges or to become a provider on a managed care panel, negotiating a managed care contract or your salary as an associate in a practice, or even applying for a loan. The only way to enter this kind of game is with a strategy directed at changing the game itself. For example, when I watch the NCAA basketball tournament, I see "underdogs" win using strategies directed at changing the game of the opposing team – after all, the top seeds have already demonstrated that they will win if allowed to play their own games. This same strategy can work equally well in the game of business.

According to "The Right Game" authors Brandenburger and Nalebuff, changing the game requires changing one or more of a game's five elements – the players, added value, rules, tactics, or scope. Focusing on these five elements will provide a framework and a systematic way for developing a strategy for changing the game. Start by asking the questions: "Who are the players? Who should the players be? How will the other players react to my actions? How much value do I bring? How valuable am I to the other players? What are the boundaries? If the other players are expanding boundaries into my area, how do I expand into theirs?" The most powerful aspect of this process is the fact that simply by entering the game, you change it. Any physician who has been first to challenge a prevailing "conventional wisdom" understands how significantly s/he changed the game just by entering. Knowing that your entry automatically changes the game can build a level of confidence that will take you quickly to the next level. Just be certain to take steps that assure your entry creates a win for other players as well as yourself.

The strategic options in the "game" of business are far greater than those of board or card games. We use tactics in both types of games; yet, our strategies for the two are very different. Because we can't change the boundaries or rules in a card or board game, our value remains constant throughout. If we lack the necessary piece to win a game of chess, we are in trouble. In business, however, when we consider a "piece" to be essential to reaching our goal, we can change the game by acquiring that piece through strategic partnerships – or, if we have access to capital, we can purchase it. Without knowledge of the strategy of Game Theory, it is difficult to recognize which pieces are missing – or why they are necessary to our goal. This, perhaps, is the key difference between the game of business and traditional games: in business we can change the game. While changing tactics is common to both, in business we are free to change the boundaries, rules, added value, and players. This opportunity often leads our thought process in new directions – ones that more consistently arrive at the goal of everyone winning – something we should all be striving for.

Chapter 3

Think Like an Engineer

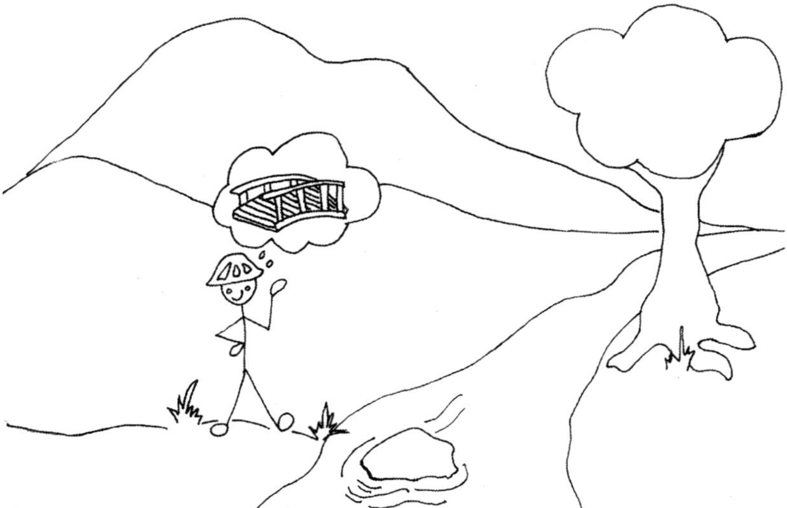

Why Engineering Is the Key to Improving Quality in Medicine

Quality is consistently mentioned as a goal of every change proposed for healthcare delivery; yet, few physicians understand the definition of this term as it is applied by employers and third party payers to the practice of medicine. Some physicians argue that they provide a higher quality of care than others and, therefore, should be paid more for their care; however, they are unable to demonstrate what it is that sets their care apart as being "of higher quality" – why it should be considered to be worth more. John M. Burns, former Vice President and Medical Director for Honeywell, Inc., summed up what large purchasers of health care products define as quality: "Quality in health care should be defined in the same way that all services and products are acquired, on the basis of the specifications of the purchaser."

When higher quality cars began arriving in the United States from Japan, people could "see" the difference. The quality of a service, however, is less easily defined than the quality of a product, and in medicine, quality is especially difficult to "see". As John Burns stated, in highly competitive businesses, the customer is the one who defines "quality." The same will be true for medicine. This means that quality will be defined by all of the following "customers": patients, employers, government, and other third party payers.

At one time, quality was defined as the absence of defects. In today's more competitive markets, quality has become the basis of competition, and achieving it requires more than an "absence of defects". In their 1991 book, *Quality or Else*, authors Lloyd Dobyns and Clare Crawford-Mason define quality as, "a better way of producing goods and services, a way that eliminates waste, gives employees pride in their work, and keeps the customer coming back for more. As you produce quality, productivity automatically goes up and costs automatically go down." This definition is one that is equally useful as it pertains to the delivery of health care, especially since doctors "compete" on the basis of both price and quality.

Good treatment outcomes are what doctors and patients perceive as quality, and this is not in conflict with a statistical measure of quality. Once a majority of doctors are able to agree upon a desired outcome, that outcome can be quantified in terms of how consistently, and at what price, it is achieved. Achieving the desired outcome consistently and at a minimum cost becomes quality treatment. The fact that a "world renowned surgeon" performs a procedure at a "world class hospital," is irrelevant if a "lesser known" doctor at a competing institution can achieve the same, or better, outcome consistently and at a lower cost.

The key to improving consistency, and thus raising quality, is to standardize process tasks. The McDonalds Corporation is a useful example of effective process standardization. While McDonald's may not deliver your idea of the best hamburger in the world, the company has determined the quality level of the hamburger it wants to achieve and has implemented standardized processes that consistently deliver this pre-defined quality. Jet Blue is another company that has been well served by its use of standardization. When Jet Blue was a startup airline, its goal was to do a better and cheaper job than its competitors, and to achieve this goal, the company focused on standardization. One of Jet Blue's strategies was to fly the same model of plane for all its routes, thus making it possible for pilots and crews to handle any flight, maintenance to be expedited, and errors to be kept to a minimum. Creating this type of standardization – in both clinical and business processes – which achieves consistent, superior outcomes, can also help a medical practitioner achieve better results while also lowering costs.

The term "customer focus" is often used when defining quality in medicine. Doctors think that customer focus simply means that they should care about their patients and render the best level of care they are capable of delivering. This, however, is *expected* doctor behavior. Quality care and customer focus go beyond this. Any doctor who participates in a contract or network is expected to be well trained and render compassionate, high quality care; this is the *entry level* necessary just to "play the game." Customer focus in medicine does not refer to these expected, entry-level attributes; rather, it can be measured statistically by cycle time (the total time a patient spends in the treatment facility). Patients value their time, and when they encounter a medical practice that recognizes this value and provides quality treatment, they perceive a total quality practice. The primary patient complaint regarding HMOs has not been about the quality of care received, but about access to that care and the amount of time spent in the facility after arriving at the appointed time. Doctors who are able to reduce cycle time will be supplying the most efficient care – the kind of high quality and cost-effective care that is valued by patients. The first step to achieving this higher level of quality is to identify inefficiencies in your practice's current business processes.

Think Scientifically When Creating Business Processes

We all know how important the grasp of basic scientific and mathematical principles is to learning the practice of medicine. Doctors need a thorough understanding of these sciences not only for practicing medicine but also for enabling continuous growth – being able to evaluate and employ any new diagnostic and/or treatment processes as they are introduced. Practitioners realize that procedures are constantly changing and that they will need to "keep up". Some treatment procedures learned in medical school ten or twenty years ago could even be considered malpractice today! Many doctors, however, do not realize that what is true for the medical procedures of their practices is also true for the business component; business processes too must be continuously monitored, updated, and made more efficient. Fortunately, the same basic sciences doctors have studied in their medical training can be applied to evaluate business processes as well.

In a doctor's office, medical treatment procedures, unlike business processes, are under the direct supervision of the physician throughout regular business hours. For this reason, they are easy for him/her to manage and change and are, thus, usually of high quality. Managing business processes, however, is difficult for many doctors. The typical practitioner has been offered little business training in medical school, and compounding this obstacle is the fact that a practice's business processes are "out of the doctor's sight" during normal business hours, with the doctor usually being unaware of their progress. Because of this, s/he experiences difficulty in supervising or changing them, and they can easily spiral out of control. It is important for a doctor to understand and become more involved in monitoring these constant, underlying business processes because an efficient, well-run practice allows the doctor more "patient time," has patients who are more satisfied with their treatment, and achieves a higher collection ratio.

Despite the fact that doctors are well versed in scientific laws that can be applied to create efficient workflow in a medical practice, they often create business processes unscientifically – processes that often defy the laws of physics. Because the high cost of practice overhead is due in large part to the inefficiencies that are created by the resultant poor processes, fixing them is the most important thing a doctor can do to increase the quality of patient care, raise levels of patient satisfaction, lower overall costs, and increase the profit of his/her medical practice. As they have done with medical treatment, doctors must learn to apply scientific laws to the business processes in their practices, keeping in mind that these laws remain "relatively fixed," despite a constantly changing economic environment.

Let's begin by reviewing the scientific principles that are critical to keep in mind when making business decisions. Prior to examining cycle time and determining how to reduce it in your practice, you must first understand how statistical fluctuations, bottlenecks, and wasted activities combine to increase the cycle time of processes, thus creating poor quality and high costs. This will make it easier to understand how correcting these problems will lead to your desired goals of higher quality and lower costs.

Finding Bottlenecks in Series Processes

I still remember my first childhood encounter with a set of decorative holiday lights. I had difficulty understanding why one entire strand of bulbs wouldn't light when they were plugged in. When I asked my parents to explain, they informed me that some of the strands were wired in series and some in parallel. I discovered that if one bulb in a series strand didn't work, none of them worked. On the other hand, if one bulb in a parallel strand burned out, the remaining bulbs would light, making it obvious which one needed to be replaced. I wondered why anyone would buy a set of series lights. The answer given me by my parents was that the series-wired ones were cheaper, presumably because they were easier to produce.

Even as a child, it seemed to me that the small cost savings offered by the series lights didn't offset the frustration experienced when they were needed and didn't work. The cost in time and aggravation incurred when searching for a burned out bulb seemed greater than the price differential of the two types of strands. If the lights didn't work when they were needed, they were worthless, and in this sense, the series lights were actually more costly. Just think of the advantage a set of parallel lights had over one wired as a series! In a series strand, each bulb had the potential to control all the others. When a strand of 100 bulbs didn't light, finding the burned out bulb required a tedious trial and error process, and if more than one bulb were faulty, it became almost impossible to find the defective ones.

Without realizing it, doctors have constructed many of their business processes just like the bulbs in the series-wired lights – as dependent series of events. The slowest step in each process (the bottleneck, burned out bulb) "limits" the efficiency of the entire process, and this limitation lowers quality and increases overall costs. This bottlenecked step in a medical business process can be as difficult to find as it is to locate a burned out bulb in a strand of series-wired lights. Complicating this problem even further is the fact that many of these series processes in a medical practice are interconnected, enabling a "burned out bulb" in one process to affect seemingly independent processes elsewhere. These "burned out bulbs" have the potential of controlling the quality and productivity of the entire practice and, thereby, the profit too.

Basic scientific principles related to "flow" are represented in this example, and they can be used to help us understand and fix many of the shortcomings in the processes we use everyday. Recognizing and understanding two important concepts illustrated by the shortcomings of series lights can help to explain why it is often difficult to find and fix problems that make our business and clinical processes less efficient and more costly than they should be.

The first critical concept to be aware of is that "fixing" any activity in a dependent series, other than the bottleneck, adds cost without improving the process as a whole. Fixing a non-bottleneck step is no different than replacing a bulb in a series strand that is functional but does not appear to be so because another bulb has failed. It is easy to see that any time or money spent replacing these “working” bulbs improves nothing but does add cost. We spend a great deal of time and money “fixing” just this type of thing in our practices, offering little to nothing in the way of results.

A second significant concept to be learned from this example is that you can lessen the effects of a bottleneck by "paralleling" around it. Just as with the lights wired in parallel, this will *always* improve the entire process. As we will see later, the concept of "paralleling" around a problem has powerful applications to many current cost and efficiency problems in medical business processes. Most important to understand is that a process constructed in parallel from the beginning will always be better than a process designed as a series.

Note that most "traditional" computer processes currently being utilized by medical practices are outdated, automated, dependent series processes that have simply been moved from paper into computers. These "new" computer processes are exactly the same as the old paper ones except that the bottlenecks are now hidden from sight “inside” a computer. It is no wonder that automation often makes things worse! Implemented correctly, however, automation can be used as a powerful tool to help us improve our workflow.

We must look for opportunities to use computers creatively – to "parallel" around bottlenecks in our processes. An example of someone outside of medicine who develops parallel processes to improve “work flow” is the freeway designer – a person who helps drivers bypass bottlenecks on highways by adding parallel lanes. Computer networks can offer medical practitioners this same kind of opportunity through the addition of remote terminals. These terminals serve as a software program’s “additional lanes” – an opportunity to bypass work “holdups” – bottlenecks. Computers also perform any bottlenecked activities faster and, if needed, continuously. This helps a practice to “keep up” with work as is it generated. The place to begin managing bottlenecks is to determine which “bulbs” have burned out and then "create" parallel processes around them, speed them up, and/or keep them working full time.

“The Hike” Bottleneck

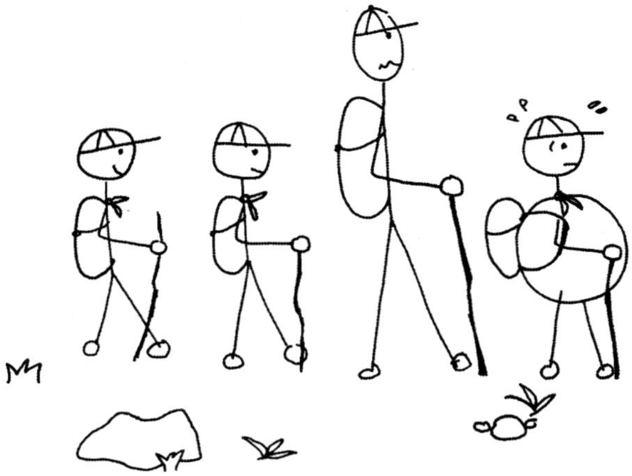

In his book, *The Goal,* Ellyhou Goldratt illustrates the combined impacts of bottlenecks and variation through the example of a Boy Scout troop's ten-mile hike. The scoutmaster in this example calculates that if each of his scouts covers an average distance of two miles, per hour, the ten-mile hike will take the entire troop five hours to complete. When his troop uses the entire five hours just to reach the halfway point, he is puzzled. What was faulty in the scoutmaster’s “scientific” evaluation? What had gone wrong?

The hike wound along a narrow trail that required the troop to walk in a single file line. The scoutmaster observed an interesting pattern develop as the hikers progressed – groups of hikers began to form, with spaces between them. The largest group accumulated behind an overweight hiker named Herbie.

As the line continued to lengthen, the scoutmaster could no longer see the boys at the front of the line and became concerned. He relayed a message to the front, asking the leaders to stop and wait for the remaining scouts to catch up.

When all the hikers had caught up with the front of the line, the scoutmaster asked that, going forward, they walk faster and attempt to stay together. They resumed the hike, but at this point, the path widened, and the faster hikers were able to pass the slower ones, eventually leaving Herbie at the end of the line. There were no longer groups of hikers accumulating along the trail, but the line began to lengthen at an even faster rate than before. The scoutmaster again relayed a message to the front of the line, asking that everyone maintain the current order and stop, in a group.

He then asked all the scouts to take hands and reverse the order of the line, putting the slowest hiker at the front and the fastest in the rear. When they resumed hiking, Herbie was at the front of the line, and the troop stayed together in "tight formation" for the remainder of the hike.

This example teaches many scientific concepts related to work flow, each of which can be of use when forming a framework for analyzing and redesigning key processes in your medical practice. The observations that the scoutmaster made throughout the hike represent statistical phenomena present in each process within a practice. Understanding and applying the principles behind these phenomena can be powerful tools for lowering costs, increasing productivity, and improving quality in any practice.

In the above example, the scoutmaster's goal was for the entire troop to arrive at their destination together. There was no advantage to having the fastest scout arrive first. In the initial phase of the hike, small accumulations of faster walkers grouped behind slower ones. We can consider these slower walkers "bottleneck hikers." There were several of these bottlenecks when the hike was in a single file series, and they were easy to spot because of the clusters of hikers behind each of them.

Bottlenecks of this type are also easy to spot in a manufacturing process. They appear as accumulations of "work in process" stacked in front of "bottleneck machines." When we evaluate the scheduling process of a medical practice, these bottlenecks show up during the busiest hours of practice in similar form – as "lines of people" waiting at the front desk and/or multiple phone lines placed "on hold". When examining a paper process, such as medical insurance billing, these bottlenecks show up as stacks of insurance forms, or other papers, on someone's desk. The introduction of computerization only makes them more difficult to detect because, as mentioned earlier, these backlogs are now hidden inside the computer and can be found only by developing reports capable of spotting them.

In the second phase of the hike, the line continued to lengthen, but with no separate groups of hikers. There were no visible bottlenecks. This is like the medical insurance process within the computer. There are no visible stacks of paper indicating bottlenecks; however, even though the bottlenecks are no longer "visible", they are there, just as before. As with the series-wired light example, there is one bottleneck that is controlling the speed and efficiency of the entire process, no matter where that bottleneck is located. In this phase of the hike, the primary bottleneck is still Herbie – he is just less noticeable now because he is located at the end of the process and is not perceived as impeding the speed of the other hikers.

The key to having this entire group complete the hike faster is to figure out how to make Herbie faster. The scoutmaster can employ a technique used successfully by both manufacturers and businesses to speed up processes; he can speed Herbie up over the short term by *eliminating waste*. This could be accomplished if Herbie were to remove his heavy backpack and distribute its contents amongst his fellow hikers. Over the long term, however, Herbie can only become faster by getting in shape (making him more efficient), and this takes time. It is important to note here that getting an inefficient office process into "shape" also takes time.

In the third phase of the hike, Herbie leads the troop, and the line proceeds slowly; however, it does stay together. This actually creates a better process in the sense that, in this order, the line is now easier to manage. In business, less need for management translates into lower costs. This does not improve the overall efficiency of the process, but it does lower the cost and complexity of management supervision – the principal focus of downsizing in corporate America. Also, when the bottleneck is located at the front of a process, the problem becomes more obvious, making it easier for everyone to focus on finding solutions for its elimination.

It is critical to recognize that no matter where Herbie is located in the line, *he* controls the time it will take for the entire troop to reach its goal (the *cycle time*). At this point, an attempt to increase the speed of the troop is a waste of time and effort if it is focused on any hiker other than Herbie. Because this one bottleneck scout controls the process for the entire troop, eliminating any other bottleneck first will not alter the cycle time. Similarly, any attempt to increase the efficiency of a process in a medical practice is a waste of time and money if it is not focused on the current primary bottleneck. Doctors are often surprised when they invest time and money "improving" their practices and don't see these investments show up on the "bottom line". These practitioners are getting the wrong scouts "in shape". They need to reevaluate their strategies and look for their Herbies.

The premise of Deming's theory of Continuous Quality Improvement (CQI) is that we need to make all of our "Herbies" faster – always focusing on the next Herbie as we improve the current one. If Herbie were to join a health club over the summer and lose weight while gaining strength, it is likely that he would no longer be the troop's primary bottleneck. The next slowest hiker would then become the new bottleneck, and following the reasoning of CQI, the scoutmaster would now work to "improve" this second slowest scout. Employing a policy of CQI in your medical practice means that you will always be looking for the next Herbie in your practice and working to "fix" him.

Variance: the Invisible Bottleneck

A question still not fully answered regarding Herbie and his fellow scouts is why it took five hours just to arrive at the halfway point when, averaging their individual speeds, it seemed they should have completed the entire hike in five hours. Later, when he analyzed their progress, the scoutmaster realized that this hike was composed of a dependent series of activities. If each scout averaged two miles an hour, he sometimes walked faster (say, 2.5

mph) and sometimes slower (e.g. 1.5 mph). This fluctuation around the average is referred to as *variance*. When all the variances (the pluses and minuses) for an individual hiker are taken into account, he shows an average speed of two miles an hour. The scoutmaster had incorrectly assumed from this calculation that the individual variances would average out evenly for the entire troop over the length of the entire hike.

The reason that these statistical fluctuations do not average out for the entire troop is that the hike is a series of dependent activities. Each scout's ability to walk faster than his average is, at times, constrained by the speed of the person walking immediately in front of him; and yet, there is no constraint on his, or any other hiker's, ability to walk slower than average at any given point in the hike. It is impossible for the variances of the entire troop to average out in the same way that they would for an individual hiking by himself. What happens is that all of these negative variances accumulate throughout the entire process (hike) and an *accumulation of slowness* results.

It is important to understand that a similar “accumulation of slowness” is unknowingly designed into every business process in our practices, and just as in the example of the hike, this accumulation is beyond the direct control of the employees working within specific processes. This is the reason that most office processes take many times longer to complete than their designers had originally intended, even when they are functioning “perfectly.” Unfortunately, those who design processes typically blame poor performance on the employees using them rather than on the processes themselves. Poor results are an indication to them that employees are simply not trying hard enough and that they need to work harder – something that will not actually improve or change an inefficient process.

All of us have experienced a manifestation of this "accumulation of slowness" on freeways. The traffic in front of our car often comes to a complete stop for no apparent reason. The actual cause might be an accumulation of negative fluctuations initiated by a car slowing (not necessarily stopping) far ahead. Resultant negative variances accumulate throughout the “system” until, at some point along the freeway, traffic comes to a complete stop. Understanding the reason for this type of obstruction has powerful applications to solving many front and back office workflow inefficiencies in a medical practice.

Understanding the way a freeway functions can help you to evaluate your business and clinical processes because the same strategies used to facilitate flow on a freeway (adding parallel lanes around fixed structural bottlenecks, quickly removing "temporary bottlenecks" caused by traffic accidents, and carpooling to reduce the number of cars on the road) can be effectively applied to alleviate "flow" problems in a medical practice. The problems of a freeway are more visible; yet, if you understand them, you will be well on your way to understanding and solving the problems that are "hidden" in your business processes.

Let us examine the billing process in a medical practice. Assume that this process consists of ten linked steps – though it actually can have many more. The starting point of the process is "marking a superbill," and the end point is "depositing a check." Similar to the hike, the process is not over until the entire "batch" is completed. If we were to measure the average time it took to perform each of these ten steps, total these times, and then compare this total with an actual measurement of a complete billing cycle for one sample insurance form, we would be likely to find that the entire process for this sample actually took ten to twenty times as long as might be predicted from the sum of the measured individual steps. If any "one-time" problems are encountered along the way – such as an absent employee or a "computer glitch," the process will be even more extended. While employees within the process can work to reduce or eliminate "one-time" problems, they have no control over the accumulation of negative variances (common problems) that regularly occurs within the process. Common problems are often invisible, and it takes statistical methods to find and reduce them.

As is the case with slowing caused by bottlenecks, the slowing created by an accumulation of negative variances adds cost and reduces the effectiveness (quality) of an entire process. As you will recall, creating a parallel process can ease the bottleneck problem by increasing capacity at the bottleneck point. We can also reduce problems caused by negative variance and can accomplish this by eliminating waste – any unnecessary steps present in a process. Elimination of a superfluous step reduces both the time needed to perform that specific activity *and* the variance associated with its performance. Eliminating wasted steps translates into being able to do a better job, in less time, with fewer employees! For example, when wasted steps are eliminated from a billing process, it can be completed faster and more effectively using fewer people. As a result, the cost of salaries is reduced, and the collection ratio is increased – both results that lead to an increase in profit.

When unnecessary steps in a process are eliminated, many related, unnecessary "handoffs" amongst staff are also eliminated. The indeterminate length of time inherent in these handoffs creates variance within a process, with the amount of time that can elapse at each handoff sometimes being considerable. Significantly, this time is "invisible" – it is certainly rarely tracked or measured. These "handoff delays" in the billing process can result in "Accounts Receivables" ranging from 30 to well over 150 days – a predicament that has a substantial negative impact on the collection percentage. Eliminating these unnecessary handoffs speeds the billing process and shortens the time that accounts remain in Receivables – again, resulting in a higher collection ratio.

As in the example of the hike, assume that "getting there together" is always an important goal. In an office, it is not important how long it takes to complete each individual task – such as filing each chart or entering the data necessary to begin the billing process. What is important is the amount of time required to complete the entire process – the cycle time. A "filing job" is not complete until *all* charts are filed, insurance cannot be billed until *all* data is entered, and the day isn't finished until all patients are seen.

To reduce cycle time, it is important to recognize that employees tend to focus on their individual cycle times – the time that it takes them to complete their own tasks within a process, but they also need to understand cycle time as seen from the patient's point of view. Staff members do not "see" the patient's total cycle time because the tasks that others do which complete the process are out of their view. Once they have completed their individual tasks with the patient, they consider the job done. Patients, on the other hand, see cycle time as the total amount of time it takes for all tasks relevant to their visit to be completed. From a patient's perspective, a "ten minute appointment" with the doctor includes the time it takes for him/her to be acknowledged on arrival, checked-in, moved to a treatment room, examined by the doctor, sent for additional tests, receive treatment and instructions, scheduled for a return appointment, checked out, and have a prescription filled. A focus on reducing this total patient time – cycle time – leads to customer satisfaction. Patients appreciate the experience of visiting an efficient, well-run practice – one where the waits are short and the treatment quality is high.

When you begin to make changes in your practice, it will be important to occasionally step back and re-think the points made in our examples of the series lights, the hike, and the freeway. Experts whom you might hire, including computer specialists, often do not understand these principles as they apply to the workflow in a medical practice. You must be able to evaluate technology (or any other device that is touted as being capable of improving your productivity or cutting your costs) from the standpoint of, "Will this eliminate my primary bottleneck?" – and because eliminating wasted activities will also reduce cycle time (eliminating, too, all the statistical fluctuations that are created by those activities), we can add to our questions, "Does this eliminate unnecessary activities?" If the answer to either of these questions is, "Yes," we must learn how to, next, quantify the cost versus the benefit of making the proposed change.

Cost reduction and quality improvement are the keys to future competitiveness and profit improvement. Speeding up bottleneck steps and reducing the variance within business processes are powerful tools for both quality improvement and cost reduction, especially when applied to critical processes in the business office. The best methods for achieving these goals are improving and re-engineering processes through creatively eliminating unnecessary tasks and increasing the capacity of bottleneck tasks.

Uncovering Hidden Waste in Your Practice

Following bottlenecks and statistical fluctuations, waste is the next most important cause of poor quality and high cost in any business.

As mentioned earlier, eliminating wasted activities also eliminates the fluctuations associated with those activities. Waste can be defined as any activity that does not add value for the "customer." In medicine's case, the term "customer" includes patients, employers, referring physicians, the Government, and Managed Care Organizations.

Detecting waste is critical to a practice evaluation because reducing waste will improve productivity far beyond what cost savings alone can accomplish. It has been found that service quality is inversely related to the level of waste. Eliminating waste not only makes an office more efficient, it lowers costs and improves the quality of the medical service provided.

When attempting to identify waste in a service business, several obstacles stand in the way. First, waste is not easily recognized because it is usually disguised in the form of extra "process" steps, all of which appear necessary. Second, and more insidious, many wasteful and obsolete business practices are still being advocated by "experts."

I began the search for waste in my office in 1989 when I innocently picked up a medical record and asked, "Why do we file insurance forms in the patient's chart?" The answer was, "In case we need to re-submit the insurance. Plus, we need a record of it." My next question was, "Don't we have a record of the insurance form in the computer which we could generate if we needed to re-submit a claim?" The answer was, "Yes, but it is easier to do it this way." I then replied, "But this process requires that you separate the copies, locate the chart, transport the chart, punch holes in the insurance form, open the chart, insert the form, and then re-file the chart."

Simple math showed me that this was, at least, a nine-step process that had the unpleasant side effect of creating unnecessarily thick charts and over-crowded shelves. I then asked, "Do we file a copy of the superbill in the chart for the same reason?" The answer was, "Yes." I then inquired, "Isn't this information also stored in the computer?" Again, the answer was, "Yes." Because the superbill was not filed in the chart at the same time as the insurance form, I deduced that I had now identified eighteen wasted steps. Add another five steps for the EOB and every other useless piece of paper that found its way into the chart. The clincher was that when I pointed this out, I was told that we didn't have a problem because we had hired two additional full-time employees to do the filing! This simple exercise identified two problems: 1) because we did not trust our computer, we ran a parallel paper system and 2) it is difficult to distinguish productive from nonproductive work.

To carry this example further, the chart that I had picked up belonged to a diabetic patient who had come to the office for routine preventative care visits every six weeks over an eight-year period. When I calculated how many wasted hours had been spent filing useless paper in this one chart over the course of those eight years, the total was 11 hours and 56 minutes – probably more time than I had spent treating the patient! This turned out to be only the "tip of the iceberg."

My next mission was to follow the movement of this chart through the office over the entire course of a single patient visit. First, it was "pulled" the evening prior to the visit and transported to the front desk. There, it was opened, a blank treatment sheet inserted, and a date stamped on the treatment sheet. When the patient arrived on the following day, it was moved to the end of the desk to signal that the patient was waiting for a treatment room. The chart was then transferred to the back office and later placed in a “slot” to signal that the patient was ready for the doctor. The doctor then transported the chart to the treatment room where notes were recorded in it before it was carried to the billing desk – a considerable distance away. The chart was then placed in a "to-be-filed" pile, all of which would be re-filed at a later date. This process consisted of thirteen steps, twelve of which were waste. Over eight years, this chart has gone through 2,496 wasted steps. As you might expect, this was not the end.

I always manually marked this particular patient’s diagnoses and services on superbills. Later, another person would enter this data into the computer – duplicating at least three of the steps I had already completed – and, significantly, creating opportunity for errors and delays. When the patient would leave the office, she waited to speak with the receptionist at the front desk in order to schedule her next appointment. To accomplish this one task, the receptionist had to stop, put the phone on hold, inquire as to the nature of her next appointment, schedule the appointment, and fill out an appointment card. She might even continue a conversation with this patient while the patient phoning in to the office waited on hold. A person in the back office who was already familiar with this patient's most current clinical needs could have appointed her more efficiently. The wasted step total for this one chart over a period of eight years is now 2,912. This figure is relatively small; patients requiring more complicated services present even more opportunities for wasted steps.

Because so much waste of this type is present in most practices, solving "the waste problem" presents a practitioner with numerous opportunities for decreasing costs and increasing quality. This also presents the opportunity to turn wasted activity time into productive work time.

Total Quality Management – The First Step Is to Ask the Right Questions

The term "Total Quality Management" (TQM) combines all of the efficiency concepts discussed in this section: bottlenecks, variation, and waste. TQM has come to be associated with the return of U.S. manufacturing firms to new competitive levels. Despite the potential for similar gains in the service sector, the health care industry has been slow to incorporate TQM principles. Successfully applied to a medical practice, these techniques can lower costs without lowering quality. No matter what course the health care industry ultimately takes, higher quality and lower costs are becoming increasingly important.

One reason the health care industry has been slow to adopt TQM is that the diverse concepts of this discipline are difficult to apply. Also, a quality product is more easily defined than a quality service. Some TQM concepts include: teamwork, cross-training, continuous learning, continuous improvement, elimination of waste, elimination of bottlenecks, customer focus, employee autonomy, cycle time reduction, and group problem solving. Many of these concepts will be effective only when applied in an environment of "commitment" rather than the old fashioned environment of "control". This is especially important in a medical practice. Because doctors are occupied treating patients and have little time to supervise or "control" employees working in the business office, these employees must be capable of acting independently, and this requires that they be committed to what they are doing.

The most important use of TQM is identifying actual problems so that proper solutions can be implemented – a "proper" solution being one that raises quality and lowers costs. Because identifying the correct problems is critical to making successful decisions, this needs to be re-emphasized. Identifying the "wrong" facts will lead to the wrong solution just as the wrong surgery, even if performed well, will lead to a bad result. Business schools teach case studies of companies that have instituted TQM methods. One classic case is that of the Florida Power & Light Company (FP&L). A June 1992 article in the management magazine, *Across the Board*, uses FP&L as its example to illustrate the problem of focusing on the wrong facts.

FP&L leaders felt they had been successfully implementing TQM principles and were preparing a visit to their mentor, Kansai Electric, in Japan. The company's leaders were excited, feeling they had solved a serious problem – they had greatly reduced the time it took to repair boiler tube leaks – thus minimizing the time the utility would be shut down each time a leak occurred. They were hoping to impress executives at Kansai Electric by demonstrating to them how quickly they were now able to repair leaks.

When FP&L representatives arrived in Japan and asked the executives at Kansai how long it took them to repair leaks, Kansai executives did not seem to understand the question. At first, thinking that their question had been lost in translation, the FP&L executives continued to restate it in different ways. Eventually, the interpreter, translating a reply from the Kansai executives, asked, "Why do your tubes leak?" Kansai had found a method for preventing leaks; they had no need to shorten the repair time!

Similarly, medical practitioners spend a great deal of time and money fixing the wrong problems – their "leaks" – because they are focusing on the wrong facts. Individual practices typically piece processes together over a period of years, "fixing" various problems as they occur. Often, because the individuals "engineering" these processes are focusing on the wrong facts, the result is an accumulation of processes that are rife with waste and bottlenecks.

The procedure that practices go through when "computerizing" an office offers a common example. Many doctors spend a great deal of time and money integrating computer systems into their practices, with little resultant increase in quality or lowered costs. The problem is that the processes programmed into these computers are seldom ones that have been improved; they are simply the practice's same old paper processes merely being performed on electronic screens.
In my practice, the search for the "correct facts" began when I asked the question, "Why do we file these in the charts?" This question led to the discovery of an important bottleneck – the paper charts themselves. Another of our office bottlenecks was created by the fact that data from superbills was not entered into computers on the day of treatment. We asked the question, "How do we eliminate this delay in data entry?" Kansai executives might have asked, "Why do you need to enter this data twice?" After all, the doctor has already marked the diagnosis and charges; once should be enough. As we analyzed other processes in our practice – from scheduling to people movement – we made similar discoveries.

It is current practitioners, attempting to make a living in today's highly competitive environment, who have the most to gain by applying TQM and re-engineering principles and methods. As soon as they begin to do so, they will be well on the road to finding the answer to such questions as, "Why do your tubes leak?" Preventing problems is the foundation of cost-reduction and quality improvement, and while physicians understand such a principle when applied in a clinical setting, they seem to have a mental block when it comes to applying this same principle to operational and financial issues. Let's take a look at some more examples utilizing the engineering principles outlined above to get you thinking about how you might apply these concepts to improve your medical practice.

Addition by Subtraction: Simplify Your Processes

When contemplating ways to stimulate growth in their practices, most doctors automatically expect that they will achieve growth by *adding* something. Hoping to grow profit, their strategies are typically focused on finding ways to increase their patient numbers and/or supply more services. Marketing budgets are focused primarily on strategies designed to accelerate growth in patient volume. While it makes sense for a practice to focus on ways to increase referrals – especially in the early years of growth – strategies for mature, or busy, practices should not be limited simply to "adding more." When we examine revenue growth from a different perspective, we can see that, sometimes, the appropriate strategy for growth may be just the opposite of "adding something."

Growing a business that provides services is quite different from growing one that manufactures products. The delivery of services requires people, and there are ultimately upper limits to the amount of output that each person is capable of providing. The author of an article in the April 2010 issue of *Harvard Business Review* entitled "The Acceleration Trap," presents an interesting perspective of "companywide burn out problems" associated with growth. He identified three types of destructive activities encountered by companies as they reach maximum capacity: 1) employees are overloaded because they have to perform too many activities, 2) employees are asked to do too many types of activities, and 3) there is constant change. Instead of asking employees to suggest additional initiatives to improve their companies, the author suggests asking employees which of their current activities and projects they believe should be terminated. He cited one example where, simply by asking, "What should we stop doing?" employees came up with 540 ideas (three times the annual number of suggestions for new-product ideas). These suggestions led to the termination of 40% of the company's projects, resulting in reinvigorated employees and an improved bottom line. Based on this research, when seeking growth in your practice, part of your process should be to regularly ask yourself, your partners, and your staff the following question: "Which of our current activities and projects would we start now if they weren't already under way?" Any activity or project that does not make this list should be considered for elimination.

An apropos quote that sums up this "less is more" approach comes from Douglas Adams, author of *The Hitchhiker's Guide to the Universe* and *The Salmon of Doubt*. When asked about creativity and innovation, Adams responded with, "Some of the most revolutionary ideas come from spotting something old to leave out rather than thinking of something new to put in." This is an important concept to keep in mind when your goal for growth is "achieving greater profitability." Typically, when a physician sees a staff person who is temporarily idle, s/he often feels the need to give that person "something new" to do to keep him/her busy, feeling that – after all – staff are not being paid just to "sit around" and "do nothing." The problem in this instance is that the physician should be looking for results rather than visible activity – especially activity that adds nothing in the way of generating better outcomes. Most of the time, this "keeping busy" activity is simply "wasting time," which has the impact of lowering both productivity and employee morale – a lose-lose outcome.

Similar to the above example in which the termination of 40% of its projects was the appropriate strategy for one company's growth, from my experience, there is no question that at least 40% of the tasks being performed in the typical medical practice are unessential and should be eliminated. Such streamlining not only reduces costs that add no value but also speeds up the time it takes to complete and capture the value of essential projects. Regardless of what growth-focused ideas you come up with in the future, make sure that your strategy includes determining not just what to add but, equally important, what to subtract.

Eliminate Process Side Chains

Every financial or treatment outcome achieved by a medical practice requires completion of a multi-step process. The quality of these outcomes, as well as the cost of producing them and the revenue generated by them, is determined by the workflow design of these processes and the volume being moved through them. The more efficient the workflow, the better the opportunity to leverage technology, office staff, and office space. A practice can attain dramatic improvement in both profit and treatment quality by focusing on the workflow steps required to achieve desired outcomes. Many of the tasks performed in healthcare processes are unnecessary, and some are performed in the wrong order, or at the wrong locations – resulting in constraints on efficiency, productivity, and performance. Some "necessary" process steps are lost in the shuffle, "fall through the cracks," and are lost to follow-up, resulting in medical errors, high costs, missed charges, low collections, and poor financial and treatment outcomes.

To gain an appreciation of just how workflow impacts quality, cost, and revenue, it is necessary to understand variability and the impact that it can have on cost, quality, and the workflow of a medical practice. Let's take a look at the workflow steps in the "simple" process of answering a phone call at the receptionist's desk. A typical example is as follows: A patient calls, and the receptionist answers. The patient asks, "What is my balance?" The receptionist answers, "Your balance is ten dollars." This is a fast, simple, three-step process, and *Flowchart A* is a process "map" of this workflow.

Flowchart A

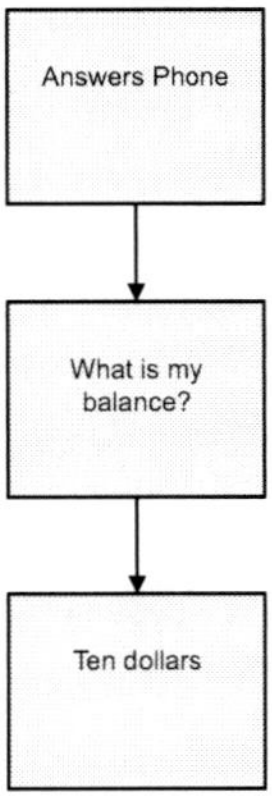

Flowchart A represents the ideal workflow, but "ideal" is rare in the typical medical practice. The potential variables that can disrupt this efficient flow are numerous, and all of them result in higher costs and lower patient satisfaction. What if, for example, the receptionist is unable to answer the patient's question? This changes the workflow. S/he must now either leave the front desk to search for the information – putting the caller on hold and the leaving front desk empty – or page and interrupt another employee in order to transfer the call to him/her so that s/he can answer the question. This "new" workflow (depicted in *Flowchart B*) demonstrates the phenomenon that I refer to as "growing a side chain." The side chain "growing" to the right is a visual representation of the extra, and often avoidable, tasks that result from variation. The randomly occurring extra steps added by this *variation from the norm* create cost and quality problems because they add time without adding value (taking time away from productive tasks), require more than one staff person to perform (avoidable handoffs), and unnecessarily delay outcomes. This type of variation lowers employee productivity, increases the need for hiring additional employees, and leads to a decline in patient satisfaction as waiting time increases.

Flowchart B

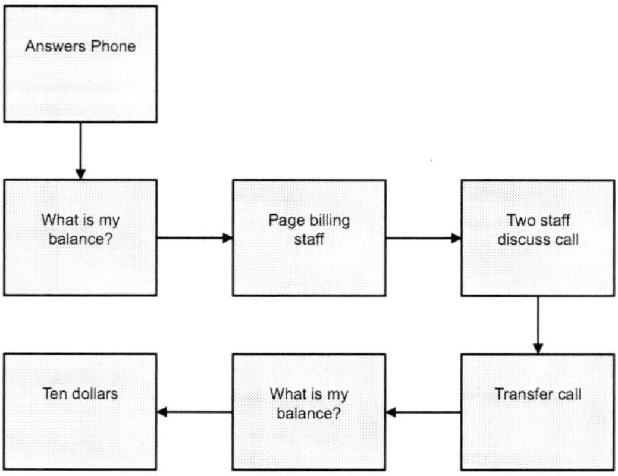

There are a number of potential variables at each process step. The next possible variable in our example occurs if the receptionist cannot immediately locate the necessary information while the patient is on the phone or if, when attempting to transfer the call, the person being paged is occupied or unavailable to receive the call. Now, a message must be taken and transferred to the staff person doing the billing so that the work can be followed up at a later time. This adds future work and creates the opportunity for the follow-up work to fall through the cracks. Up to this point, both the patient and the receptionist have invested time, and no result has been achieved. When the biller picks up the message, s/he may need to retrieve the chart to obtain the information before returning the patient's call. Once the information is located, the biller places the call. What happens, however, if the biller cannot find the chart or, when returning the call, finds the patient unavailable? This often results in a game of telephone tag. As can be seen in *Flowchart C*, the side chains for this relatively simple task continue to become ever longer and more complex.

Flowchart C

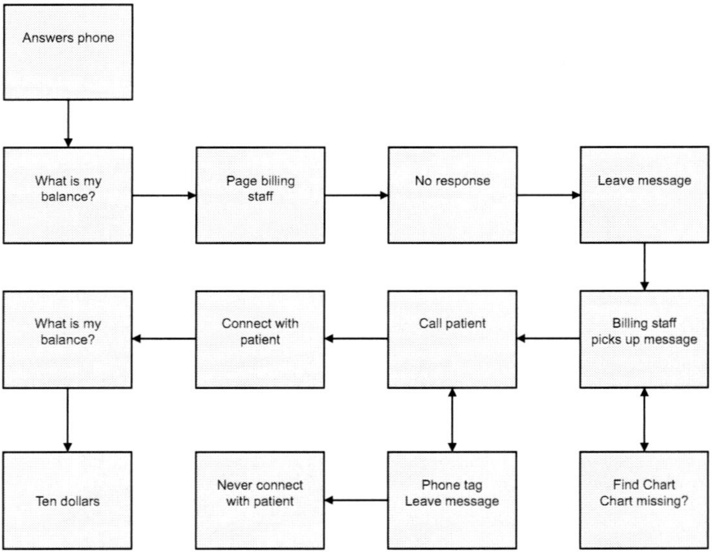

Each decision point, each handoff to another person, and each piece of work set aside for completion at a later time creates this potential for variation – setting the stage for errors, unnecessary work, prolonged delays, and the possibility of data being lost or work never being completed. Each time this occurs, cost is added, quality is decreased, and completion of a task is delayed. All of this, in turn, delays the outcome of the entire process. Points at which variation can occur are similar to crossroads where different paths can be chosen. On a process map, these new paths appear as side chains (depicting extra work) – which eventually circle back to the original flow. While side chains cannot be totally avoided, at least 80% of them can, and reducing their frequency will dramatically improve the efficiency of workflow and increase productivity. Side chains occur randomly, hundreds of times a day, in every process and in every area of a practice. Furthermore, many processes are connected, allowing variation in any one to impact the others.

Returning to our original example, it usually takes less time for the first person encountering a task to complete it than it does for that person to refer the task elsewhere. Faster and better service is rendered when the receptionist can say, "Your balance is ten dollars" rather than, "I don't have that information. Let me transfer you to the insurance department." In this case, the receptionist must then complete the transfer process by interrupting the person doing the billing. When we require two employees to "do the job of one" it is always more costly and takes more time. There is no benefit to saving one employee's time if transfer of his/her work increases someone else's time for achieving a delayed outcome. It is always better for all doctors and staff members to complete any work as they go along – as long as this does not take away from their productive time. It is also better for a patient to receive an answer on the first phone call or from the first employee s/he "interrupts" while in the office.

If I were to ask a staff person, "How long does it take to find a patient's medical record?" a typical response might be, "Between thirty seconds and a minute." This might represent the average range of time required to find a chart, but what if it cannot be found on the first or second attempt? This is a common occurrence in medical practices that do not use an electronic medical record, and it serves as a good example to understand how unnecessary variation increases costs and lowers quality. In this case, the medical record is not "lost," it could be in the insurance office, on the doctor's dictation machine, or even in the trunk of the doctor's car. If a medical record cannot be located, the staff person will continue looking. Perhaps, after five minutes, s/he will begin interrupting others, possibly with a second staff person joining in the search. At this point, there are technically two staff members "not working." At some point, if the medical record cannot be found, the patient is eventually brought back to a treatment room with the doctor being given a temporary chart containing only blank sheets of paper. In this example, the unnecessary variation has caused two staff members to be idle, other staff – or even the doctor – to be interrupted, the patient to wait an extra twenty minutes, and the doctor to see the patient with no prior history available. Not only does this lower the quality of care, but this visit is going to require more of the doctor's time because s/he needs to re-take the patient's past history. This example demonstrates clearly how low quality can lead to high expenses.

Now, imagine what happens when several types of variation occur simultaneously. This is what happens at those key times in a day when everything seems to fall behind, leading to chaos. For example: a chart cannot be found for the patient who is checking in at the same time that a call comes in, needs to be transferred, and the person who the call is being transferred to is not at his/her desk. Another call comes in while the receptionist searches for a missing chart, and a person is waiting on hold for the biller – who is "missing" (most likely looking for a chart). While this is happening, a patient arrives at checkout, wanting to pay her balance and make an appointment, but her charges and appointment routing slip have not yet arrived at the front desk (the doctor has gone on to the next patient without marking her charges). As you can imagine, the side chains of this workflow diagram increase rapidly in both number and length. The space that it would take to diagram this chain of steps would take several pages in this book. The big problem is that in many practices, these side chains are accepted as "normal" and may even be intentionally "hardwired" into existing workflow and computer systems. This type of workflow becomes the rule rather than the exception, and it usually arises due to insufficient information or the inability to transmit information from the point of service. Just imagine the possibilities for increased variation as groups and networks grow larger!

No workflow design is ever 100% ideal. The hope is for the 80:20 rule to prevail. That is, for 80% of the potential side chains to be eliminated (with only 20% remaining). The opportunity for major improvement lies in the fact that in many cases, these side chains are growing from workflow steps that are unnecessary! Removing wasted steps eliminates not only unnecessary work but also 100% of the side chains associated with that work. All side chains resulting from certain process steps (such as finding charts, entering charge slip data, or transferring sticky note messages) are 100% correctable because the process steps themselves are unnecessary and can be eliminated. The challenge lies in being able to step outside of the processes (or office policies) with which you have become comfortable and determine which of the ones you are using have been designed in ways that *guarantee* inefficiency and variation. Only then will you be ready to consider changes.

The 20% exceptions mentioned above – the 20% of side chains that serve useful purposes – might be initiated when patients call with complex questions requiring special knowledge – such as something about Medicare rules or the results of lab tests. These are the types of calls that should be transferred to staff members – or the doctor – who have the expertise to answer "specialty questions." Conversely, there are many questions thought to require a doctor's or back office staff person's expertise that can actually be answered at the front desk, or by any staff member who happens to be idle at the moment a call comes in or a patient in the office asks a question. In these cases, the information required to answer that question must be immediately accessible to the person at the location where the call is received or the question asked. A practice must also have appropriate training and office policies in place – giving staff members who answer the phone or who are asked questions in the office accurate information and authorization for answering these questions.

Another important point to recognize is that as a practice becomes busier in the course of a day, more decision points arise at which a staff person must make a determination as to the urgency of a task (versus creating a side chain by transferring it to another staff member or putting it off until later). Urgent tasks include such things as: a ringing phone, patients who arrive to be checked-in and out, and charts that must be tracked down in order to treat patients. Less urgent work can be put off. Don't confuse "less urgent" with unimportant. Usually, it is the most important and most strategic types of work that can, and will be, put off – sometimes indefinitely. In a busy office, the functional Murphy's Law is that: If it can be put off, it will be. This work usually includes such things as strategic planning, reviewing management reports, updating codes, training staff, and implementing new technology (such as an electronic medical record).

Obviously, if technology is going to assist a doctor in making improvements in his/her practice, it must be applied in a way that improves workflow through elimination of tasks or side chains. This won't occur automatically – even when the "best" technology is used; simply having the best is not enough. In fact, technology is often used in a way that actually adds to the number and length of side chains – increasing the odds of losing more information to follow-up. The process of streamlining workflow has both technical and non-technical components. In addition to eliminating steps and side chains, the doctor and staff must determine what type of information to deliver, where it should be delivered, the form in which it should arrive, the training needed to access and use the information, and the type of office policies regarding access to information that must be put in place. If any one of these issues is not thoroughly thought through, there is potential that workflow will not be improved, even if all the others are in place. For example: a practice might adhere to an office policy that requires the receptionist to transfer all billing questions to someone else, even when that receptionist has the time and technology available to her/him by which s/he could quickly access the information him/herself and respond to the question.

Whenever a decision point exists in the workflow, the questions to ask are: "What type of information needs to be accessed at this point? What training (or cross-training) is needed in order to be capable of accessing it? What authority is needed? How should information arrive – as a pop up note or through a rapid search mechanism? Also, what questions or transactions (the "necessary" 20%) should be referred elsewhere?" If a process has the potential of developing five different side chains and each can grow even longer under certain conditions, eliminating four of these chains (80%) represents a major accomplishment. Technology can then be applied to a well thought out process, enabling certain types of controls and "smart" decision support services that will further reduce the frequency of the 20% of "acceptable" variations.

The more sizable a practice's patient volume or number of process steps, the greater the likelihood that variation from the norm (side chains) will occur. Variation is possible at each step in every process within a medical practice, and its presence always has a negative impact on both cost and quality. An efficient workflow design is one with the fewest number of steps necessary to get the job done properly. With an efficient design in place, a process is continuously improved by staying focused on speeding up the necessary steps and reducing any existing variation. This will always lead to processes that produce the highest quality at the lowest cost.

Consider the process steps a doctor completes when seeing a patient. They might include: examining the patient, taking a history, ordering tests, educating the patient, dispensing information, writing a prescription, discussing a return visit, marking a routing slip, marking a charge slip with the diagnoses and charges, receiving messages, sending reports and/or a referral letter, and transferring information to the staff regarding the need for treatment authorizations or scheduling procedures. Imagine the number of possibilities for variation along the way – or putting off work for later – in the course of a busy hour or a busy day. The ideal is for a doctor to stay caught up throughout the day and complete tasks in a timely manner. Physicians must develop a new mindset that sees side chains as unacceptable. Once a practice is focused on workflow and the amount of time it takes to complete a process, it is on the path to improving quality, increasing productivity, and lowering costs.

Error Reduction Speeds Processes and Reduces Costs

The front desk of a busy medical practice can appear chaotic, often resembling complete pandemonium. At multiple times on a typical day, patients are waiting in line to speak with the receptionist who is engaged in checking people in, answering the phone, and making return appointments – all at the same time. For most practices, this "check-in" area is the point at which all patient demographic and insurance information is entered into the database. Because of the time pressures, the phone distractions, and the "in-person" interruptions that this person handling the data entry process can experience concurrently, the odds for making mistakes can soar.

"Small" mistakes typically made at the front desk are generally tolerated because they are seen as an unavoidable consequence of this turmoil. The problem with tolerating this imprecision is that these small errors add up over time, and they become costly because of the many man-hours required to "find and fix" them at a later time – resulting in lower collections and necessitating an increase in staff numbers. While no process is ever 100% error free, high error rates should never be accepted as "normal." With proper focus, a busy practice can reduce the number of errors made during the check-in process, dramatically impacting both practice quality and profitability.

Errors made at check-in create extreme variance in the length, cost, and end result (collections) of the billing process. When a patient checks-in at the front desk, the ideal process is as follows: the staff person 1) inputs the demographic and insurance information correctly, 2) collects the patient's co-pay, 3) submits the insurance, and 4) receives a check. This flow is ideal because it includes only three major steps, the practice's collection ratio is optimum, staffing ratios can be kept low, and little backlog develops.

When a mistake is made, however, the process changes to the following: the staff person 1) inputs demographic and/or insurance information incorrectly, 2) does not have the information required to collect the co-pay, 3) submits the insurance form, 4) receives a rejected claim, 5) sets the rejected form aside for later follow-up, 6) retrieves the patient's chart, 7) identifies the error or omission, 8) contacts the patient to obtain the correct or missing information (which can require leaving a message, often resulting in a lengthy phone tag process), 9) retrieves the accurate information, 10) re-enters the correct data, 11) re-submits the insurance form, 12) mails an invoice for the co-pay, and finally, 13) receives the check.

What is potentially a three-step process, completed in one day, can easily become an eleven-step process, extending over many weeks and necessitating additional steps – thereby creating further backlogs and delays that result in lower collections and the necessity of hiring more staff.

The error rate typically increases as a practice becomes busier. A billing staff's first priority is to "stay current" (focusing on today's claims), and because of this, they tackle the growing "do-over pile" only when they feel that they are "caught up." The typical practice eventually hires more personnel for dealing with this growing backlog, and the size of the staff hired to tackle it can become needlessly large, especially in group practices.

Research has shown that companies operating at a one to five percent error rate (3-4 sigma) spend 25% to 40% of their revenues finding and fixing problems whereas companies operating almost error free (6 sigma) spend less than 5% of their revenues performing the same tasks. I have encountered many group practices that have an error rate much higher than five percent and would think they were doing well if they could reduce this to one percent. In reality, one percent is still unacceptable. These excessive costs that medical practices typically pay for finding and fixing errors, are in the form of higher staffing ratios (costly payrolls), decreased productivity (lower revenues), and lower collection ratios.

How can we alleviate this potential inefficiency and reclaim the consequential lost profit in our practices? A friend of mine who works for Hughes Aircraft once told me that when something was done incorrectly at Hughes, the engineers would say, "There is never time to do it right, but always time to do it over." This statement hints at our problem as well as its solution. As doctors, we know it is better and less expensive to prevent disease than it is to treat it. The same holds true for dealing with the clerical errors in our practices.

The money saved by not hiring enough staff with sufficient time to enter data correctly and check for errors before moving forward is an illusion. When we "save money" in this way, we in turn lose far more income due to the copious amount of staff time required to find and fix mistakes at a later time and the accumulation of delays (leading to lower collections) created by these mistakes. We need to hire and cross-train a sufficient number of staff to handle the front end of the check-in process in order to prevent errors and avoid backlogs.

We will need to improve our error rates in order to improve the quality of our practices and increase our collections, but this will happen only when improving them becomes a high priority.

Lowering these rates requires that the doctor create new reports for measuring the number of errors. Without such reports, there is no way of knowing what a practice's error rate is, where the errors are occurring, and whether their number is increasing or decreasing.

As has been noted, the majority of data input errors can be avoided by providing front desk staff with sufficient time to enter information correctly and to double check for omissions. "Extra" time can be created for this purpose by increasing the number of staff and/or by increasing efficiency – implementing strategies such as reducing the number of interruptions and eliminating unnecessary tasks. If you are in the process of increasing the number of "front desk" staff in your practice, keep in mind that it makes the most sense to add personnel at the initial check-in point than to add more of them "downstream" – where they will spend time finding and fixing errors. When errors are decreased at the "front end" of the billing process, backlogs are reduced, and the cycle time is significantly shortened – resulting in better cash flow and higher collections. With error prevention as its focus, a practice can reduce the "big effects" of "small" errors.

Chapter 4

Satisfy Your Customers

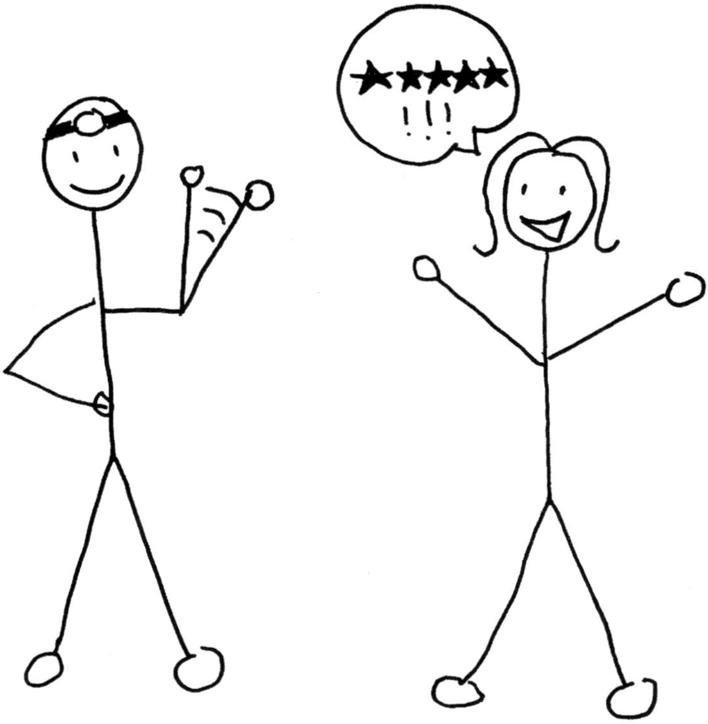

The Importance of Customer Loyalty

"How Golf Went off Course" was a featured article in the April 2, 2007, issue of the *Wall Street Journal*. The author caught my attention with the following: "The game has tried hard to draw new players, but it may have missed a bigger opportunity – getting more rounds out of its most avid golfers." He went on to explain that while golf's costly external marketing efforts had attracted new players, a much larger number of previously avid golfers were exiting the game, and an editor's note stated, "If golf spent more time doing things to make life easier for its fervent followers – such as keeping the costs down and speeding up play – it would reap the benefits." This advice stimulated my thinking about the importance of patient retention in medical practices.

Doctors who are just out of residency and establishing their reputations need to attract new patients, and it is important that they have external marketing plans for this; however, practice growth (in terms of the annual numbers of new and return patient visits) generally follows an "S" curve – growing slowly the first few years, accelerating for a period of time (which might continue for many years), and eventually hitting a peak at which the annual number of total patient visits levels off. At this "leveling" point, the practice volume is in equilibrium, adding approximately the same number of patients each year as it loses to attrition. This is when most doctors who are aspiring to grow their practices perceive that an increase in the number of new patient visits will be the solution to their "volume problems" – leading them to focus the majority of their time, effort, and money on external marketing.

A doctor wishing to grow or prevent a decline in patient volume beyond this equilibrium point can learn from the example of the golfing industry, s/he needs to focus on more than external marketing and attracting new patients. Loyal, existing patients are often overlooked as a significant source of opportunity. I believe that doctors will find the patient volume obtained from a well thought out internal marketing program – directed at patient retention – will go beyond that which these doctors are seeking through traditional external marketing. In fact, an "internal" patient retention plan simultaneously offers external marketing (through existing patient and doctor referrals), resulting in an influx of new, as well as retention of "old," patients.

If practice growth is your long-term goal, following the advice of Ed Zore, CEO of Northwestern Mutual Life Insurance is a worthwhile path to follow. When asked for tips on growing a business in a mature market, his advice was as follows: "Respect existing clients. Treat them well. Don't add new customers at the expense of losing loyal ones. You keep and grow market share by delivering value over the long term."

Why Do Customers Leave?

A survey on "why companies lose customers" conducted by the American Society for Quality (ASQ) found that only 18% are "lost" for reasons not directly under the company's control – as when a customer moves. The majority of customers are lost for reasons that *are* under a company's control, with 68% leaving because of the service provider's attitude of indifference and 14% because of dissatisfaction with the product or service. Consider the following benchmark statistics gathered from a broad mix of industries: 1) the average company loses 10% of its customers each year, 2) the process of acquiring new customers can cost six times more than that required for satisfying and retaining current ones, 3) a 2% increase in customer retention has the same effect on profit as cutting costs by 10%, and 4) studies have shown that a 5% reduction in customer attrition can increase profits by 25% or more. Similarly, a strategy focused on "preventing" patients from leaving a medical practice is preferable to one focused primarily on attracting new patients who are not yet loyal to the practice. In fact, if a doctor is not continuously focused on patient retention as his/her practice grows, the number of patient defections will increase as the practice becomes "busier," making it even more difficult to attract new patients.

Based on the results of ASQ's survey, there is no question that an effective internal marketing program must include a major focus on doctor and staff "attitude," which is essential both to retaining existing customers and attracting new ones. Many companies focus so much time and energy attracting new customers that they create the appearance of being indifferent to existing ones. This perceived attitude encourages existing customers to leave. If you have ever purchased a cell phone contract, you have most likely experienced this phenomenon. How often have you seen a promotion from your own phone provider offering a better deal to its new clients than the one you have (such as offering free phones and/or rebates), and when you ask for this same "deal," you are told that it is not available to you as an existing customer? This approach builds zero loyalty and, in fact, encourages clients to turn to competitors. Believe it or not, some doctors do this same thing; they are so focused on attracting new patients that they appear to be giving them priority over established ones. Similar to the phone company example, existing patients will definitely sense that new patients are getting a better "deal."

Consider the approach taken by United Airlines when it was close to bankruptcy with the company's future existence in doubt. Management made the decision to focus on retaining its existing clients, especially the ten percent who were considered frequent flyers and accounted for fifty percent of revenue. I am one of United's frequent flyers, and in spite of delays, cancellations, and a host of customer service problems throughout this difficult time, I remained loyal to United because of its highly visible efforts to retain my business. This type of strategy can build customer loyalty for any business. It builds word-of-mouth referrals and gives existing customers a compelling reason to say something good about the company. I am sure that you have all heard medical practice management speakers relate that dissatisfied patients are more likely to tell far more people about their bad experiences with a practice than satisfied ones are to tell about their good experiences. Simply adjusting your attitude and focusing on factors that affect patient retention can shift this leverage from negative to positive.

How Can I Increase Customer Loyalty?

While ASQ questioned clients from a variety of industries when conducting its "satisfaction and loyalty survey," a comprehensive survey specific to medical practices, conducted by Press Ganey Associates of South Bend, Indiana, was published in the December

4, 2006, issue of *AMA News*. The company polled and ranked the responses of 1.4 million patients who were treated at 5,400 sites nationwide. The results, listed in *Table 4.1*, are ranked in the order of "satisfaction traits" most likely to foster patient loyalty to a medical practice.

Table 4.1: Top Reasons for Patient Satisfaction and Loyalty

1	Sensitivity to patient needs
2	Overall cheerfulness of the practice
3	Overall care received during visits
4	Comfort and pleasantness of exam rooms
5	Waiting time in exam room before being seen by a care provider
6	Amount of time the care provider spends with patients
7	Care providers who make an effort to include patients in treatment decisions
8	Instructions given regarding follow-up care
9	Convenience of office hours
10	Promptness of returning phone calls
11	Concern (by nurse or assistant) shown for patient questions or worries
12	Helpfulness on the telephone
13	Length of wait before going to an exam room
14	Patients' confidence in the care provider

If you believe the adage, "A problem well stated is a problem half solved," then a simple awareness of the ranking of the concerns listed in *Table 4.1* and their impact on patient retention will solve half of your retention battle. Knowing that the majority of factors affecting patient retention are directly related to perceptions of the attitude of the doctor and/or staff tells us that a good place to start "internal marketing" is to identify which of the fourteen items from *Table 4.1* might be creating a perception of indifference for your patients.

Fortunately, many negative perceptions can be changed relatively easily. The items listed in *Table 4.1* show us that seventy nine percent of the changes we need to make can be implemented fairly quickly. Fifty percent are likely to be directly, or indirectly, related to patient perceptions of "an attitude of indifference" or feelings that they have received insufficient information to meet their needs (items 1, 2, 7, 8, 10, 11, and 12). Providing adequate information should increase patient compliance and, correspondingly, improve outcomes. This will have a positive impact on items 3 and 14. If we add "convenient office hours" (item 9) and "comfort and pleasantness of exam room" (item 4), we now see that eleven of the fourteen items (79%) listed in the table can be implemented in a relatively short period of time. These changes will significantly increase patient loyalty and retention and, as a "byproduct," improve treatment outcomes. Those items requiring improved processes (such as shortening wait time in the exam room) are more involved and will take longer to implement, but technology that you already have in place should be able to help you improve these processes.

An Informed Patient Is a Happier Patient

The number of healthcare websites has exploded – mostly due to patients who are seeking medical information. Patients come to doctors seeking diagnosis, treatment, *and information*; yet, while doctors are very good at diagnosing and treating problems, many are not nearly as good at providing information. Patients often perceive this shortfall as a lack of interest from the doctor, which substantiates their perception that healthcare providers have an "attitude of indifference." Consider a classic by Charles Schultz from his *Peanuts* comic strip. This excerpt shows Snoopy lying in a hospital bed with his three brothers looking on. One asks, "How can we know if our brother is getting better if no one tells us anything?" A second says, "I think I'll go hang around the front desk … maybe I'll hear something …" When he returns, he looks dejected, stating, "The nurse is having trouble with her boyfriend, and the doctor is going to switch to a metal seven-wood." While the comic strip is funny, it conveys a negative perception widely held by patients. Patients want information, but their perception is that no one at the doctor's office really cares.

In addition to asking questions arising from natural curiosity about their conditions and treatment, patients are being encouraged by experts to question the necessity of tests and X-Rays that their doctors order. Patients have long been told that doctors practicing defensive medicine often order more tests than are medically necessary, and there is documented evidence to this effect. An interactive Harris poll released earlier this decade confirms this opinion, indicating that 80% of doctors order more tests than are medically necessary and that more than half of these tests are invasive. I don't know about you, but for me, the thought of paying for a painful test, and then later finding out that it may not have been necessary, is scary. I want to know ahead of time that the results of a test I am being asked to undergo will be of value to my treatment.

Patients don't know which tests are necessary; however, they are being counseled that because some tests may not be absolutely necessary, they should ask questions regarding any tests they are encouraged to undergo. Many practitioners react negatively to such inquiries, interpreting this as an indication that patients doubt their judgment. It is important to understand that this is not necessarily the case. Today's patient is a better-educated consumer and understands that there are important questions to ask before submitting to a test, especially if it is to be an expensive and/or invasive one. We cannot ignore the fact that patients are being educated to know when to question or say no to a test, and we need to approach this trend as a positive. Understanding that patients are being educated to question the necessity of tests, we can choose to meet their needs rather than regarding this as a challenge to our judgment.

It is best that we anticipate the questions patients may ask, including those that have to do with the medical necessity or cost of tests. This preparation will lead to our patients having a high degree of confidence in us – confidence that any test we recommend as necessary *is* necessary and will increase the likelihood of a correct diagnosis and a good treatment outcome. This preparation will also improve patient compliance with our treatment plans because it involves a patient in his/her own treatment.

Implementation of patient education can be difficult in today's environment of low fees and high volume – a time when most doctors are feeling the "crunch." Most seem to have little time to devote to this crucial matter. According to the article "Educating and Enlisting Patients," in the *Journal of Clinical Outcomes Management*, by Geoffrey H. Gordon, MD, FACP, and F. Daniel Duffy, MD, FACP, clinicians tend to overestimate the amount of time they spend "instructing" patients. According to a study cited in this article, physicians estimate that they spend an average of seven minutes educating each of their patients; yet, when followed throughout the day, with their time allocations being "scientifically" measured, the "education time," per patient, actually turned out to be one minute or less. If physicians actually did spend seven minutes educating each patient regarding his/her condition, they would achieve dramatically higher levels of patient satisfaction, and treatment outcomes would be consistently better. Unfortunately, if doctors actually did spend seven minutes educating patients, they would likely go out of business. What is difficult for busy doctors – ones who seemingly have only one minute, per patient, to devote to this activity – is coming up with a "creative equivalent" for those seven minutes of "education time."

Neil Baum, MD, a urologist practicing in New Orleans, has found one solution to this problem, something he has been using in his practice for many years. Dr. Baum has filmed five to seven minute videos in which he explains common urologic conditions and procedures, including their complications, risks, and expected post-operative courses. After examining a patient, he presents that patient with a video on his/her specific procedure/condition. The patient views this video in the treatment room while Dr. Baum goes on to see other patients. Afterwards, he returns to answer any questions the patient may have regarding the information in the video. While the patient is in the treatment room "being educated," Dr. Baum is usually able to see one or two other patients. How can others implement this model into their practices? Since effective future medical delivery will require technology in treatment rooms (for the utilization of electronic medical records), this same technology can be used to serve the parallel purpose of presenting audio-visual patient education material and, thereby, further improve treatment outcomes and physician productivity.

Video presentations can be augmented by printed educational materials and a practice website. The printed materials can be dispensed in treatment rooms or at check out, and the website can be visited in-office or at home. In addition to its being a valuable teaching aid that helps patients learn about their medical conditions, a website creates the opportunity for patients to learn about other conditions the doctor treats – conditions which an acquaintance, a friend, a family member, or even they, themselves, may have. The end result of this dissemination of information is a true win-win; the patient receives the medical information s/he is seeking, patient compliance increases, outcomes are better, patient satisfaction increases, the doctor is able to use his/her time more effectively (directing it to more productive uses), the practice receives more referrals from "better-informed" patients, and third party payers save money as a result of improved treatment outcomes. Given the positive impact that effective patient education can have on a practice, it makes sense for all physicians to incorporate educational videos or PowerPoint presentations, printed materials, and websites into their practice routines.

Doctors who use electronic medical records have a "leg up" in their efforts to customize information for individual patients. As the doctor writes an electronic prescription, the EMR software automatically checks for allergies and drug interactions, produces a legible prescription (with the correct dosage), supplies written instructions that augment anything the doctor has already discussed, and supplies printed information explaining the patient's diagnoses, treatment, and follow-up. If the patient has any questions after s/he exits the practice, many of them are best handled by e-mail. The point is: if you are focused on eliminating your patients' perception of "indifference," there are numerous ways that technology can be employed to accomplish this without requiring more physician or staff time.

Listen to Your Patients

An article by Meredith Levine that appeared in the June 1, 2004, *New York Times* entitled, "Tell the Doctor all Your Problems, but Keep it to Less Than a Minute," provides insight into the perception that doctors don't care and that patients are not informed. According to the author, within 18 seconds of a patient's explaining his/her problem to a physician, the doctor interrupts. This certainly conveys a lack of interest. This article goes on to state that when it comes to informing and educating patients about their conditions, only 15% of patients actually understand what the doctor tells them, 50% are uncertain of what they are supposed to do when they leave the office, and 33% forget what they have heard by the time they get home. It is no wonder that it is difficult to achieve a high degree of patient compliance. According to Wendy Levinson, M.D., Vice Chairperson of the University of Toronto's Department of Medicine, this perceived "lack of interest," coupled with poor patient compliance, results in poor treatment outcomes. According to Dr. Levinson, "A feeling they were not listened to and didn't have the doctor's full attention" is a common theme in malpractice lawsuits.

One useful benchmark that signals whether or not a doctor is listening to his/her patients is the number of times a day s/he hears the dreaded comment, "Oh, by the way doctor ..." just as s/he is finishing with a patient and is about to exit the treatment room. This is the point in time at which the patient brings up a whole new problem – one that has probably been bothering him/her for a long time but has not been acute enough to warrant taking a day off work to see a doctor. If you happen to be one of those doctors who interrupts patients within 18 seconds of their telling you about their conditions, any time you think you may have "saved" is an illusion. Studies have found that in most cases, when a doctor allows a patient to continue talking, 150 seconds is the maximum amount of time needed for that patient to express all of his/her concerns. Interrupting actually increases the amount of time spent with the patient, presents an opening for the "Oh, by the way" question as the doctor is exiting the room, leads to a perception that the doctor doesn't listen, and increases the likelihood that the treatment outcome will be sub-optimal.

The Waiting Room: a Patient's Worst Nightmare

Two significant areas of concern to patients are: 1) How quickly will I be able to access the doctor when I have an "emergency"?

and 2) How much time will I spend waiting once I arrive at the doctor's office? Being aware of and dealing with these two issues related to "time" can provide a medical practice with strategic advantage. Many doctors recognize this and refer to same day access and short waits as "magnates for attracting new patients." If your practice is seeking to attract new patients, or retain existing ones, addressing these two patient concerns should be a significant part of your focus.

How much time does a "fifteen minute" visit with the doctor actually take? The answer to this question varies considerably, depending on whom you ask – patients or physicians. Editor, Marianne Dekker Mattera's "Memo from the Editor" column in the July 7, 2006, issue of *Medical Economics* is entitled, "Your 15 Minutes, My Day." In this memo, Mattera examines a typical patient visit that from the doctor's perspective, is represented by a fifteen minute time slot in his/her schedule. From the patient's perspective, however, this "time slot" is longer – possibly even consuming an entire productive day. As a general rule, any doctor who understands this "time issue" from the patient's perspective is likely to achieve better treatment outcomes and greater profitability.

In this *Medical Economics* column, Mattera describes the office visit of a patient who has a fever, in conjunction with a red, hot, edematous leg. The patient's wife (actually, Marianne Dekker Mattera herself) feels that her husband may have cellulitis and wants to schedule an appointment early the next morning so that he can be seen before the weekend (this is a Thursday evening). The particular practice that she calls has the habit of not taking calls before 10:00 am, even though staff arrives at the office much earlier. After leaving a phone message – which is not returned – Marianne arrives at the office in person at 9:15 am, scheduling the appointment for 11:45 that same morning. She and her husband arrive early (at 11:15 am) but are not taken into the treatment room until 12:45. The doctor does make a diagnosis of cellulitis and writes a prescription, but he also wants to send Marianne's husband to an imaging center to rule out DVT. The receptionist calls the imaging center, is able to make an immediate appointment, and the patient goes directly over. There, the wait is not long, and DVT is ruled out; however, because a "swollen gland" is noted on the scan, the referring doctor now wants the patient to return to his office for blood work. By the time blood work is completed, the prescription picked up at the pharmacy, and the patient arrives home, it is 4:30. This is the "fifteen minute" appointment from the perspective of Marianne and her husband.

This patient's experience is not as uncommon as it might seem. While an appointment with a doctor may not require a patient's entire day, a typical visit occupies a great portion of the day, and a "fifteen minute appointment" requires substantially more of the patient's time than the doctor and his/her staff might realize. Obviously, we do not have direct control over the extended time that may be needed outside of our own offices; however, "sensitivity" to the potential for this extended "outside time," improving the wait time for initial access to our practices, and lessening patient waits during our portion of the treatment *are* things within our control, and all will go a long way towards improving our patients' treatment satisfaction, our treatment outcomes, and as a result, the profitability of our practices.

Quick patient access and short waits require streamlined business operations. Implementation of new operations necessitates significant planning and, sometimes, lengthy processes which are often undertaken as a result of "philosophical changes" or "attitude adjustments" by the doctor and/or staff. If you plan to undertake this type of change in your practice, a good place to start is to remove all your barriers to access. For example, most doctors talk about wanting to grow their practices and attract new patients, but when patients call, it would appear to an outside observer (a role I often play) that their staffs have been instructed to "keep patients away." Patient calls are often treated as interruptions, rather than as opportunities, with some patients actually having to "talk their way" into appointments on a busy day. This is a significant barrier to practice growth. The negativity with which some doctors react when they see a new patient visit being "squeezed" into the schedule on a busy day assures that it will be even more difficult for the next new "emergency" patient to access the practice in a timely manner. New, streamlined business process will enable the efficient and effective scheduling necessary for quick patient access and short patient waits.

Consider what goes through a patient's mind when making an appointment. For starters, because of previous encounters – such as the one that Marianne and her husband experienced – the patient knows that a fifteen-minute visit might require a half-day, or more, of his/her time. Since the visit may not be as "urgent" as in this example, the patient is unlikely to make an appointment at all if s/he cannot secure a desirable time slot. The patient also knows that even if s/he manages to schedule at the desired time, it is unlikely that treatment will actually begin anywhere near that scheduled time. If they cannot secure desirable time slots, many patients end up not making appointments at all – or they go elsewhere. A practice incapable of providing same day access for existing and new patients may need to address this problem by adding another doctor, staff person, or treatment room, incorporating greater efficiency into his/her practice, or a combination of all the above. Of course, this assumes that doctors and staff first remove all of their philosophical barriers to access. If you are aware of this problem and are ready to make this change in your practice, you have already taken the crucial first step in making it happen.

Forming Virtual Groups Can Make a Patient's Visit More Convenient

In June 1997, I authored a newsletter focusing on consolidation as a key force that would shape healthcare in the future. In this article, I concluded that the optimum health care delivery model would be composed of single-specialty networks that were focused, efficient, physician-driven, and "virtually connected" with other specialty networks for the purpose of providing coordinated care. These models would deliver the best care to patients at the lowest price to payors. They would also provide providers with the highest profit margins – margins that would average as much as 30 percent more than those of traditional multi-specialty models.

In 1997, experts claimed that the jury was "still out" on the single specialty versus multi-specialty debate. The one "advantage" claimed for multi-specialty models was that they, somehow, would be better able to coordinate total care, with the ultimate goal of delivering "seamless care." It is hard to imagine that the more complex, multi-specialty, group could ever be the most effective model, especially considering the 30 percent cost and efficiency advantage that single-specialty groups typically achieve. Additionally, many multi-specialty groups have yet to provide additional convenience, even when the specialties are all "under one roof." For example, if a patient sees a doctor at a hospital clinic or a large academic medical center and, during that same visit, needs x-rays, lab tests, and an appointment with another specialist, the experience of that patient is often no different than if he or she were scheduling each of these appointments at different hospitals. Although the departments are all "under one roof," they are neither integrated nor coordinated in a seamless fashion. But how can independent, single-specialty groups, given this one perceived disadvantage of not being able to coordinate care, actually deliver care more seamlessly than multi-specialty groups? Reframing the question from the patient's perspective opens up new possibilities. The question now becomes, "How can I, the patient, receive seamless care?" At first glance, the difference between the two points of view seems subtle, but this will point the way to solving the question of how independent, single-specialty groups can collaborate to deliver seamless, high-quality, cost-effective, "multi-specialty" care.

A single-specialty group does not have to determine how it will deliver seamless care. Instead, it can focus on integrating and governing its own members in a way that achieves the greatest internal efficiencies, reduces treatment variation amongst the member doctors, and thereby, renders the best quality care. This requires that each practice first be made optimally efficient and then integrated into an efficient, virtual, single specialty network. All doctors would use the same software, including an electronic medical records package containing treatment protocols upon which all doctors have agreed. If desired, these single specialty networks could then group with networks from other specialties, forming "virtual" multi-specialty networks by "connecting" their single specialty networks to a "central office" from which treatment would be coordinated. In this way, each patient's care would be "seamless."

Reframing questions from the patient's perspective assures that solutions will be customer-focused. Since these virtual, multi-specialty models are created by digitally "connecting" efficient, physician-driven, single-specialty models, they are not only best for doctors, they also deliver the greatest value to patients and payors – a true win-win-win scenario.

The Ethics of Profiting from "Premium Services"

In an effort to improve customer satisfaction, some doctors charge a fee for "premium service." Rather than judging this approach on its merits, critics have questioned its ethics. There may be good reasons why charging for premium services is or is not a good strategy, but ethics are not the relevant issue.

Premium pricing is based on services that are focused on convenience; it has nothing to do with the quality of the medical care rendered. In order to put this in an understandable perspective, consider the following example: Three patients drive to a doctor's office. When each arrives, s/he has the following parking options from which to choose: 1) $1 metered street parking – two blocks away, 2) the medical building's parking, at a cost of $6, or 3) front-door, valet parking for $10. A patient who wants to save money leaves for his/her appointment a little early and happily parks the two blocks away. One who wants the convenience of being closer chooses to pay the $6 to park in the building, and a patient who is not "price sensitive" or is in a rush on that particular day may choose to pay $10 for the added convenience of valet. Does the fact that each patient chooses to pay a different parking fee for his/her physician visit (based on the value s/he places on convenience) have anything to do with ethics or third party reimbursement for the medical care s/he receives?

Now, consider the experience of two patients with the same condition who choose to see two different physicians. Patient One waits three days for an appointment, spends a total of two hours in the reception and exam rooms before seeing the doctor, and following treatment, is accorded little time with the doctor for questions regarding his/her condition. Later, when this patient calls the doctor's office with a question, the call is not returned in a timely manner. Patient Two, on the other hand, is given the option of being seen immediately, is greeted warmly by the staff upon arrival, waits only ten minutes before seeing the doctor, and following treatment, his/her subsequent questions are answered patiently and thoroughly by the doctor and staff. Additionally, Patient Two is provided with printed information and a web page to check for additional information and given the doctor's email address to use for further questions that may arise. A cell phone number to call in case any post-treatment complications arise is also provided. Under our current healthcare system, third parties pay the same fee for both services, but these patients are clearly not receiving the same service. Is this fair? Given that a patient's time is limited and that many today are demanding value added "convenience" services, is it unethical for a doctor who provides these extra, value added services to charge the patient for them?

I believe that critics are being sidetracked by the amount of money being charged by some for premium services rather than focusing on the relevant issue. Third party reimbursement is received for medical care, not convenience services. The marketplace will determine the premium services that patients will value and the amount doctors can reasonably charge for them. A patient might be willing to pay extra for short waits or quick access (value added tasks), but not for the cost of obtaining authorizations or sending out statements (non-value added tasks).

When concierge-type services were first offered by medical practices, a small number of doctors took the approach of charging an outrageously high annual membership fee to all patients wishing to remain in their practices. Annual amounts ranged from $800 to as high as $20,000. A Cincinnati doctor was in the news for charging a $1,500, per year, membership fee for same-day appointments, more face time with the doctor, prompt return of phone calls, and e-mail accessibility. Because these services are actually ones that, when offered in conjunction with enactment of efficiency principles in a practice, will reduce the doctor's costs while attracting more patients, this $1,500 fee will be unlikely to survive market competition. Efficient practices will be able to offer same day appointments as a matter of routine; however, the fact that some patients are willing to pay $1,500 shows just how much they value quick access and short wait times.

Consider a more reasonable option of a $9 premium for each office visit that includes value added convenience services that patients are asking for. Say that a medical practice's average revenue, per patient, is a low fee of $44. The new fee, which includes the $9 premium, would be $53 – increasing the total office visit fee by 20%. For a practice with a 60% overhead, adding a higher level of convenience for this small $9 premium could increase profit by 50%! This seems a reasonable amount for a patient to pay for added convenience, and it could "fix problems" at the practice level for both patients and doctors without adding to the costs for third party payers.

Another Patient Concern: How Much Will My Visit Cost?

A consumer who wants to make an intelligent economic choice must have accurate price information. You might recall a T.V. commercial that aired some time ago in which a potential customer asked a sales person, "How much is your $1,200 dollar computer?" with the sales person replying, "$1,800 dollars." Makers of this tongue-in-cheek commercial were intending to show the lack of "price transparency" in the computer industry. Today's prices for medical services are even less transparent.

Researchers examined claims data from May 2010 to May 2011, representing 82,000 employees working for small businesses in the same town. They found that some patients payed as much as 683% more than others for the same medical procedures, such as MRIs and CT scans. As the computer industry has matured, pricing has become more transparent; however, even though the healthcare industry has matured, patients still have little idea what price they will be charged for specific services. The doctors who astutely recognize that this is bad for patients and doctors alike will greatly benefit by making their pricing information more accessible to patients. If you knew that prices for the same service could vary by as much as 683%, wouldn't you want to know the price of a procedure you were going to undergo ahead of time?

Providing consumers with accurate pricing information is fundamental to success in every business; we take accurate pricing information for granted for practically every product or service we purchase. As it turns out, every healthcare reform plan that has been put forth to "fix our broken system" also recommends this need for greater transparency. Why sit on the sidelines waiting to be "forced" to provide this type of information to patients when it is in your interest as well as the interest of your patients to do so now?

The reason most doctors have taken little initiative to assure that their fee information is transparent is because they either believe this to be unprofessional or worry that patients are comparison shoppers looking for the cheapest doctor. A better argument is that it is unprofessional to *not* make price information more accessible. The reality is that, because of the huge variation in physician charges, patients are hesitant to make appointments, often assuming that fees will be much higher than they actually are. It is the "not knowing" that keeps many of them from making appointments in the first place, especially those who have high deductibles or who are paying cash – those who may very well represent the majority of future patients. If increased transparency of information makes economic sense for all businesses in all industries, why wait for it to become a requirement in medicine?

A large medical group in California caused quite a stir, making front-page news in the *Los Angeles Times*, when it made prices available to consumers on its website. Patients were now able to learn that this group's fee for a chest X-ray was $61 and that physical exams ranged from $140 to $160. Prior to this posting, patients may have thought that exams would be much higher – which does certainly occur at some offices. Armed with information from this practice's website, its patients are now able to budget for visits, knowing in advance how much they will cost.

A patient who makes an appointment for a consultation with a new physician faces constraints based on previous experiences s/he has had visiting doctors. How often does a patient come to your office and complain about the outrageous fee s/he was charged for a consultation by another doctor? This is usually followed by negative comments regarding the small amount of time the doctor actually spent with him/her. Assume that your charge is $175 for a consultation. A patient is more likely to make an appointment and pay in full if s/he knows ahead of time that this is your charge. Even if your charges are fifty percent higher than those of another practitioner in your area, a patient knowing this fact, who has been referred to you by another doctor or a trusted friend, is still more likely to choose you over the doctor who charges less. Without pricing information, a patient may fear that your fees could be "astronomical"; in this case, the possibility of the patient scheduling is reduced.

Transparency in medicine will eventually include information regarding both quality and price. Information regarding quality will be more subjective and difficult to measure, but this is the information that will ultimately enable patients to assess value. Third party gathering of this type of information is still in the early stages; yet, physicians today can begin providing information regarding the quality of their practices to patients. Traditionally, doctors have considered their personal credentials (such as education, training, certification, and hospital affiliations) to be the primary measures of quality, but patients want information regarding their own specific needs and treatment options. Supplying the type of quality information that is important to patients will help to demonstrate your practice's greater value to them and, subsequently, validate higher, but fair, fees for your services. Ultimately, information and price transparency will be required of all doctors. What are you waiting for? It makes sense to proactively take this on now.

Do You Know How Much Patient Treatment Costs?

A survey in the October 2000 issue of *Archives of Internal Medicine* showed that 80% of physicians did not know how much their patients actually paid for prescriptions. This apparent lack of concern is no longer acceptable. Physicians – the ones who write the prescriptions – have the responsibility to learn more about both the benefits and the costs of the various medications they prescribe. They have the option of recommending that patients change to equally effective, but less costly, generic or "me too" brands. The end result will be better healthcare, including increased trust of physicians, lower costs for patients and payers, and a lessening of pressure to reduce physician fees.

A *Wall Street Journal* article I read a few years ago showed how a retiree cut his quarterly prescription costs 64% (from $700 to about $250) just by "talking to his doctor." The doctor discussed how the patient's blood pressure and cholesterol medications could be replaced by cheaper, but equally effective, generic drugs. The patient saved a substantial amount of money, and his blood pressure continued to be just as well regulated.

Avoiding unnecessary treatment is also a point of concern for patients looking to save money – a concern that, all too often, is not shared by doctors. Medical doctors often have patients who arrive with conditions (such as viruses) that have no "cure" and will simply, in time, run their course. In spite of this, many doctors will order tests (just in case) or write prescriptions. Many of these tests and prescriptions are "practice management habits" that doctors have developed over the years because their patients feel that they have performed little of value if they have not ordered tests or written prescriptions. An example cited in the "Health and Family" section of the February 14, 2003, issue of the *Wall Street Journal* is of a patient who returned from a cruise with viral symptoms. The patient's doctor ordered $400 worth of blood tests. Ultimately, the virus ran its course, and the patient was better – leading him to wonder whether the blood tests had been necessary. Many such tests performed – and prescriptions written – increase the price of healthcare without adding value, and both doctors and patients bear the resultant financial burden.

Offering Convenience: Dispensing Supplies in Office

The AMA has hotly debated the ethics of allowing medical practices to sell supplies and products to patients. Doctors have argued that with their incomes declining, selling supplies and products offers them an opportunity to capture a new source of revenue. Ethics gurus argue that doctors shouldn't be selling supplies to patients because this takes advantage of a trusted relationship for the purpose of making a profit; however, neither of these arguments is relevant to the issue. Under fee-for-service reimbursement, unethical doctors have always had an economic incentive to take advantage of a trusted relationship by inflating charges or providing unnecessary services. Under capitation, the same unethical doctors have an economic incentive to withhold necessary services. Does it logically follow that fee-for-service and capitation are unethical? Whether recommending care or selling supplies, there is always an economic "ethical dilemma." The relevant issue is that an unethical doctor will do whatever benefits him/her most, and an ethical doctor will do whatever benefits the patient most; whether the doctor is making a profit, or not, is irrelevant to the discussion. In a discussion of the relationship between ethics and profit, I don't see how dispensing a medical product differs from providing medical treatment.

Take the example of a woman I know who took her two sick children to a pediatrician. That doctor prescribed a medication for both children. Upon leaving the office, the mother asked a staff member if the prescription could be phoned in so that it would be ready when she arrived at the pharmacy. The staff person informed her that she was too busy to call the pharmacy, leaving the mother to carry two sick, crying children back to the car, drive to the pharmacy, find another parking spot, take the kids out of the car and into the pharmacy, and then wait twenty minutes for the prescription to be filled. What if, instead, the pediatrician had offered this mother the option of purchasing the medication at the front desk, at the same price the pharmacy would be charging? I think that this mother would have been extremely grateful.

So, I ask: What is the ethical dilemma involved when a doctor recommends insoles, a knee brace, vitamins, skin cream, or any other product, and then gives a patient the option of purchasing them in his/her office? This is not the same as selling the patient a 'secret potion' that can only be purchased at his/her office. My opinion is that patients will see this as a superior service, providing them with a desirable benefit – especially elderly patients. Making a profit, whether it comes from clinical care or selling needed products, is irrelevant to the discussion. Other businesses would refer to this as being "customer focused" and would argue that practices providing these products deserve to earn higher profits.

In reality, suppliers have expanded their boundaries into areas that are competitive with our medical practices. Many patients opt for self-treatment, which quite often involves the purchase of an over-the-counter medication or product. If we were to recommend any of these products to a patient, believing it would be beneficial, doesn't it make sense that stocking that item would provide a valuable service for that patient? Not only is it convenient for patients to receive products or medication at their doctor's office, but the doctor or staff can also instruct the patient in the product's use in a way that is likely to achieve better compliance and optimum results. The patient can also be steered away form medications or products that may be either unsafe or ineffective.

If you do decide to dispense supplies in your practice, you may be wondering, "what products should I keep in stock?" Common sense might suggest that product displays allowing a patient to choose amongst numerous choices would produce more sales and greater profit than ones with fewer choices. A series of research studies, however, suggests that beyond a certain optimum, the presence of too many options actually hampers a buyer's ability to make a choice. Sheena S. Iyengar conducted the most dramatic of these studies at Columbia University. Iyengar's research compared grocery store shoppers who encountered two different displays of jams and jellies, one featuring a choice of six flavors, and the other, a choice of twenty-four. Even though more shoppers were attracted to the extensive display (60% versus 40%), only 3% of these customers made a purchase, while 30% of those presented with the limited display did so. The display with fewer choices produced ten times the sales of the more extensive display! You can draw your own conclusions from this study, but it certainly seems to indicate that when showcasing supplies and/or products for sale in your office, less might very well be more. Not only are you likely to achieve more sales if you use a limited display, but the display will require less space for showcasing and storage, and because inventory will be less complex, its management will require less time.

The following offers a convenient option for those who decide to dispense supplies in their practices. While having supplies on hand for a patient's convenience makes sense, a practice does not need to stock a large supply in the office. Re-orders can be filled through the practice's website or through an outside service vendor. This enables the practice to reap the benefits of dispensing medical supplies, durable medical goods, and medications, without having to purchase large quantities of merchandise, store the items, or physically dispense them. This allows the practice to "stock" its website's virtual store with items that its patients need without the hassle of creating a retail store in-office. Most importantly, this "store" is open for business 24/7.

Patient Satisfaction Surveys: An Objective Measure

Hopefully, by now you are convinced that patient satisfaction and patient loyalty should be Number One on your "to achieve" list. Experts typically recommend the use of surveys for assessing how well a practice is accomplishing this. Patient satisfaction surveys are similar to the customer satisfaction surveys used by businesses for assessing how well they are meeting customer needs and for gathering marketing information about unmet needs for which new services or products might be developed.

A flaw typically inherent in satisfaction surveys is that they tend to be long and complex, resulting in low response rates and unclear results. A recent study by Frederick F. Reichheld, author of *Loyalty Rules!* and Director Emeritus of the consulting firm Bain & Company, found that the results of such surveys rarely correlate with company profits or growth. This is a problem because the typical goal of a customer satisfaction survey is to provide information that will help a company grow and, presumably, become more profitable. While "growth and profitability" are rarely the stated goals of patient satisfaction surveys, they are targeted at gathering information useful for retaining existing patients and attracting new ones – the achievement of which leads to growth and profitability.

As a result of his research, Reichheld came up with one "solution" for the length and complexity defects of satisfaction surveys and their lack of correlation with growth and profit. He published his "solution" in the December 2003 issue of *Harvard Business Review*. Reichheld had set out to determine whether the typical list of survey questions could be reduced to a single question – one useful as a predictor of growth. There could be no solution simpler than a one-question survey, and the results would be extremely useful if they served well as a predictor of growth.

Working two years, determining how best to link survey responses to actual customer behavior, Reichheld found that the types of behavior with the strongest links to company growth were its customers' purchasing and referral patterns. Through study of these patterns, he hoped to find one question that fit each industry which would be useful for predicting customer behavior correlated with growth. What he found was a single survey question that served this function best for *most* industries. That question was, "How likely is it that you would recommend [*Company X*] to a friend or colleague?" Using a scale from one to ten for measuring responses (ten: extremely likely to recommend, five: neutral, and zero: not at all likely), those customers who selected ratings of nine or ten were labeled "promoters." Reichheld concluded that creating more of these promoters would be a sure path to increased growth and greater profitability.

Results derived utilizing Reichheld's "simple survey" can be extremely useful. Using just one question, a company can measure the number of "promoters" it has and then focus on increasing this number, with the expectation that this process will lead to increased growth and profit. In effect, the "promoters" become part of the company's marketing department, and increasing their number leads to growth and increased revenue as well as higher profit margins because the costs are zero for this important segment of the marketing department's "work."

While the results of this study may seem somewhat obvious to physicians who rely on promoters (both patients and physicians) for growth, many involved in Reichheld's research found it counter-intuitive. They had expected questions directed at product or service quality, standards of excellence, or customer loyalty to be more predictive of customer promotion. Physicians, however, know that a satisfied, loyal patient is not necessarily a "promoter." Those who refer others are more than loyal; they go a step further. In effect, these patients are putting their own reputations on the line when making referrals.

While I do not intend for doctors to scrap their current patient satisfaction surveys and replace them with single question forms, there is significant data suggesting that we should rethink the number, type, and complexity of the questions we ask on our surveys and that we should have in mind a definite purpose for the results of these surveys. There is significant data from Reichheld's study to suggest that this one question of how likely it is that the patient would refer patients to this particular practice should, at least, be included. Perhaps, it should be the first question, followed in turn, by a limited number of others – perhaps enquiring as to why the patient does, or does not, recommend the practice to others.

Keeping Your "Other Promoters" Happy: Referring Physicians

The impact of physician referrals on the growth and reputation of a medical practice is widely recognized. When a physician refers to a fellow practitioner, s/he is expressing confidence in that doctor's ability. A successful referral expands the reputations of both the referring doctor and the doctor "referred to" within the medical community. In their early years of practice, doctors typically put significant time and effort into seeking these referrals; however, as their practices become busier, they tend to take referrals for granted, assuming that they have already proven themselves to their referring doctors. While this may be the case with practitioners who happen to be close friends, it is rarely the case when the referring physicians only know the doctor to whom they are referring by reputation, referral letters, and feedback from referred patients. As a practice grows and becomes busy, a clear understanding of "referral dynamics" (especially the weight given to patient feedback), will assure that existing referrals are retained and the number of new referrals is expanded.

To increase your understanding of "referral dynamics" let us look closely at the physician referral process. A way to approach this is to look inwards and take a critical look at what goes into your thought process when you are deciding to whom you will refer a patient. Why do you continue to refer to certain doctors and not to others? An experience of mine might help you to answer this question. Several months ago, an out of town friend called and asked if I knew someone in his area for his wife to see for a foot problem. She had become unhappy with the doctor she was seeing. I made a recommendation. Recently, out of the blue, I received an e-mail from my friend's wife stating, "I saw Dr. 'X' today, and I want to thank you, thank you. I won't bore you with the details, but just wanted to let you know that I am so glad that I contacted you and that I saw a doctor who listened to me. Now I will go out on my daily three mile walk, thanks to you and Dr. 'X.'" This is the ultimate positive outcome of the referral process:

a win-win, for the patient, the referring doctor, and the treating doctor.

Obviously, an e-mail that opens with "thank you, thank you" is something that any doctor enjoys receiving; however, there are several important details in this e-mail. The significance of the message, "I saw a doctor who listened to me" is powerful; patients place confidence in physicians who listen to them. My interpretation of this patient's e-mail is that she would have sent me a grateful response even if the treatment provided by Dr. X had not helped her problem because this doctor had "listened" to her. Since the treatment did actually help, notice that *both* Dr. X and I are receiving credit for her positive experience. My reputation, as well as the treating doctor's, has been impacted in a positive way, and "all" I did was make a referral. This is an important point: every time a doctor makes a referral, his/her reputation is also at risk, based on that patient's experience.

How do we maintain and grow our list of referring doctors? Since a doctor's reputation is at risk when making a referral, s/he generally takes great care when referring and in following up with patients regarding their treatment experiences. It is in the interests of the referring doctor as well as the patient that s/he gets into the best hands possible. If the patient has a bad experience at a referred visit, s/he is likely to blame both doctors, and that referring doctor is less likely to refer to the same practitioner in the future; however, if the experience turns out to be a positive one (as in the example above), the patient gives the referring doctor equal credit, and that doctor referral relationship continues. Also, a satisfied and enthusiastic patient is likely to go out of his/her way to find even more patients to refer in the future.

As simple as this example seems, examining how you determine whom you refer to provides a sound approach for understanding why a physician might refer to you. Undergoing this process should result in an increase in your physician referrals and/or retention of your existing ones. When a physician receives a bad report from an unhappy patient, it ruins his/her day. The "income" that a physician receives for making a referral is psychic – making it very important to hear a "thank you" from the patient. Since bad reports from patients to referring doctors most often result from patient perceptions that treating physicians were uncaring and/or inattentive, you should feel confident that you are in full control of your ability to retain and increase referrals to your practice.

If you find that, as you become busier, you are becoming more complacent about your existing referrals and are beginning to take them for granted, remember that "just" getting good results is not always enough; your patients need to feel that you are listening to what they tell you. What if one of your top referral sources were to receive a bad report from a patient because you happened to be having a bad day on the day s/he came in, and because of this, you weren't a good listener? Even though that referring doctor might still believe in your abilities, s/he will feel obligated to find another doctor for that patient. If so, think what might happen to your future referrals from this doctor should this second referral happen to be a doctor who is as attentive as Dr. X in the above example? Good listening skills, coupled with effective care, will lead to maintenance of existing referral sources and an increase in new sources.

Don't Rely on Patient Feedback; Send Reports Back to Referring Physicians

On October 1, 2009, I had the opportunity of attending the Regional Health Care Leaders Summit in San Francisco. During the course of her presentation, Susan Hogeland, CAE, Executive Vice President of the California Academy of Family Physicians, cited a statistic from the Academy's database which I found to be startling: only 38% of specialists report back to referring physicians after treating the patients that have been sent to them! Isn't communication with referring physicians considered to be "good medicine" – or, at least, a common courtesy? This 38% exposes a significant "free" marketing opportunity for specialists, one which any physician could take advantage of simply by practicing "good medicine."

Many of us "older" practitioners remember the days when a physician-referred practice was the gold standard, especially one receiving referrals for complex medical or surgical consultations. Today, this is the norm. Those in the past who had physician-referred practices credited their success, in part, to the fact that they consistently reported back to referring physicians, and made personal "update phone calls" at significant points in the course of a patient's treatment. Family practitioners keep lists of specialists to whom they refer specific problems, and I believe that, over time, they narrow these lists to those who not only do good work but also communicate well.

I think the fact that only 38% of today's specialists report back to referring physicians has come about as a result of managed care with its employment of "gatekeeper" systems and "preferred providers" who happened to be on a list of contracted doctors. These systems required that patients first see their family doctors who, in turn, referred out those cases that were beyond their training or experience. In a sense, this created a situation in which virtually every patient from certain health plans who was seen by a specialist was "technically" physician-referred. Overburdened managed care specialists were faced with voluminous, unnecessary paperwork, and because of this, the referral letter slowly found its way to the bottom of priority lists.

As in all of life, what one person sees as a burden, another will see as an opportunity. Even though managed care and subsequent "replacements" have increased the amount of paperwork in a medical practice, the importance of reporting back to referring physicians has not changed. What amazes me is that I still see practices with hefty marketing budgets that do not consistently send referral letters. If you happen to be in one of these practices, let me give you four good reasons for changing your policy to one that requires you to consistently send these letters:

1) This is "good medicine" for your patient's overall health

2) Referrals are an effective way of educating other physicians as to what you do

3) Good communication is a practice builder

4) The number of scenarios in healthcare in which primary care physicians will have an impact on who receives referrals and the level of reimbursement for those referrals is growing

A great amount of uncertainty still exists regarding healthcare reform and the direction it will ultimately take; however, if we are to learn anything from the past, we should recall the early days of managed care when being totally excluded from a plan or offered a restrictive contract with ridiculously low fees was a real possibility. At that time, the specialists who were most likely to be included in plans, or most likely to receive a better-than-average reimbursement rate, were those in physician-referred practices. These doctors were on the "A lists" of the primary care physicians in their areas, and those primary care doctors wanted to assure that specialists on their personal lists were included in their referral networks. The referring physicians wanted to maintain a continuation of high quality care for their patients, and "legitimate" networks were even willing to pay these select specialists a higher reimbursement rate to assure their participation. Doctors should strive for this type of reputation; today's specialists preparing for healthcare reform should make sure that primary care doctors in their areas know who they are, what they do, and that their patients give them high satisfaction ratings. The referral letter is an effective means for conveying this information.

Being overburdened with paperwork is no longer a satisfactory excuse for failing to report back to referring physicians. Given today's sophisticated information technology, a significant portion of referral letters and "update" reports can be automated from an electronic health record without being "canned" or cut-and-pasted. Ideally, this type of reporting should be completed "as the doctor goes along" (usually at the time s/he completes the patient's medical record). Using this approach, reports do not pile up or become a burden to the point that doctors discontinue sending them. The benefit of effective communication is clearly worth the cost – most of which is your time.

The Simplest Way to Improve Customer Service

A survey conducted by the American Express, Global Customer Service Barometer during the most recent recession asked 1,000 adults, "Do businesses value consumers enough?" One would think that in a recession economy, companies still remaining in business and their employees who are fortunate enough to have steady employment would feel grateful to the consumers who purchase their products and services and want to keep them happy. In turn, it seems that the vast majority of these consumers would feel valued by the businesses they frequent. Surprisingly, American Express found that the overwhelming perception of consumers responding to this survey was exactly the opposite, with 74% responding that, "businesses these days don't value consumers enough." These same respondents went even further, saying that they would be willing to pay 9% more for excellent customer service. At this point one might ask, "What is wrong with this picture, and how am I perceived by my patients?"

Over the course of your medical career, how many articles have you read, or lectures attended, in which customer service and patient satisfaction were stressed? Whatever point of service we consider – whether it be the first phone call to the office, the check-in or check-out experience, the treatment room experience, or a phone call as follow-up to a patient visit – I think we would all agree that each of these interactions presents a doctor and/or staff member with the opportunity to secure patient satisfaction by providing excellent service – the type that not only makes patients want to return in the future, but motivates them to refer friends and family and relate their experiences to their family doctors. Given the number of articles and lectures on this topic, why is it that we still need to have this discussion? Doesn't everybody already know the importance of good customer service? Evidently not, according to this survey. The survey results tell us that there seems to be a big "disconnect" between the service quality we think we are offering and what patients perceive us as actually providing.

While some changes require a long and difficult implementation process, changing our patients' perceptions of how much we and our staff members "care" about them is something that can be accomplished almost overnight. How many times have you heard the expression, "A patient does not care how much you know until they know how much you care?" How difficult is this to achieve?

When considering patient satisfaction, I think back to my first post-residency year in Vancouver, British Columbia and the home visits I was making. I remember what a ninety-four year old couple said when I informed them that I would be returning to Los Angeles to start a private practice. They told me that I was "irreplaceable" and that I would be successful wherever I went. The husband said, "Dr. Hultman, I have known you for two years, and you are always in a good mood. I do not understand why some doctors are so nasty when it takes no more time or effort to be nice." His message has stayed with me to this day. Regardless of how busy we and our staffs might be on any given day, or how aggravating we might find some patients or healthcare "rules," the reality is that we are going to be in our offices a set number of hours each day, and while we are there, it is just as easy to be "nice" as it is to be "nasty." Not only does a focus on "friendly service" make for a more enjoyable day for everyone, it is an effective means of internal marketing which will result in practice growth and a better future – regardless of what healthcare reform we face in the future.

Doctors whose patients are dissatisfied are not in a very good position to negotiate contracts, and they are in an especially bad position to "just say no" to poorly paying ones in hopes of negotiating better fees. Patients and referring doctors will not even miss these doctors when they are gone. As data relevant to patients looking to select physicians becomes more transparent and easily available to the public, there is a good possibility that patients will avoid seeing those doctors who have low satisfaction ratings and may even leave their current care givers if they are not happy with the "service" they provide – even if, according to this survey, the doctors they will be switching to are charging higher (but "reasonable") rates. Given the size of today's co-pays and deductibles and the likelihood that many "elective" services may not even be covered by insurance now, or in the future, the amount of out-of-pocket cash payments required from a patient is expected to increase significantly. The American Express survey indicates that those patients who are satisfied with their provider's service will be willing to pay larger amounts for that excellent service. Practitioners will need to remain vigilant and maintain high quality because satisfaction ratings will become ever more critical to the success of their practices. In a world of increased transparency, patients will have easy access to information that will help them to compare providers. They will be able to find comparative fee ranges and satisfaction ratings for doctors offering similar services.

How would your practice be rated if your patients were asked a question similar to the one posed by American Express – "Do businesses value consumers enough?" Would your results be better? Placing a greater emphasis on patient satisfaction may cost you little in terms of time or money, but judging from this survey, the potential payoff could be significant. Given this survey, which indicates that many businesses have apparently lost their customer focus during stressful times, isn't this the ideal time to become proactive and make sure that your practice is offering excellent service along with its quality treatment?

Chapter 5

Retain a Smart and Loyal Staff

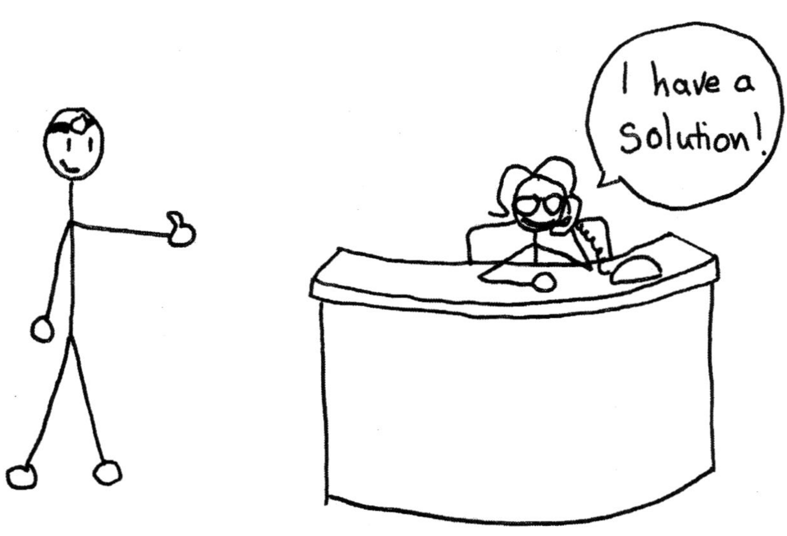

The High Cost of Employee Turnover

It is disruptive to lose a valued employee. The loss necessitates interviewing, negotiating with, and training someone new. In addition, doctors and staff must adapt to the dynamics associated with having a new personality in the office. Not only is employee turnover disruptive, it can also be costly. For all of these reasons, significant effort should be made to retain any productive, well-trained employees.

Why does someone leave a job? Usually, it is because that person is either unhappy with the salary or the work s/he is doing. Losing a productive employee to avoid increasing his/her salary typically creates a cost rather than a savings. Efforts can be made to improve job satisfaction for an employee who is unhappy with the work, and almost always, this improvement in job satisfaction increases productivity, thereby creating the means for increasing salary.

One of my first field projects in business school was assisting a member of my study group who was the general manager of an airline food service company located at LAX. This company was considering a restructure and implementation of teamwork and quality management concepts focused on reducing annual turnover rates for several job categories which were, at the time, as high as 75 percent. He recommended that the company introduce teamwork concepts, the first phase of which, upon implementation, resulted in a 36 percent reduction in the turnover rate – more than half. Application of these concepts not only made work more efficient – it was also now more "fun" for the employees.

William M. Mercer, a New York-based consulting firm, estimates that today's administrative, recruitment, and training cost per new employee in large and mid-sized firms ranges from $10,000 to $30,000. Because the administrative, recruitment, and training costs at the time of our study (1989) were calculated to be $17,500, per employee, the 52 percent reduction in the employee turnover rate resulting from the company's reorganization, saved $1,225,000 annually – an unequivocal validation of the quality improvement effort. One might speculate that using some of this "found money" to increase salaries would then have reduced turnover even more.

Applying what was learned in this exercise to medicine, we ask, "What might the cost of turnover be for a medical practice?" In a small business, the actual our-of-pocket administrative, recruitment, and training costs are relatively low, but for a medical practice, a significant cost of employee turnover is the negative impact it can have on practice productivity, efficiency, and growth. This "opportunity cost" varies dramatically amongst practices – depending on the number of staff employed by the practice and the efficiency level of its business and clinical processes.

When a practice has three employees, losing only one can make a significant impact – a staff loss of 33 percent! And, if the employee leaving happens to be a key staff member, he or she may have been responsible for more than one-third of the total staff output. When a back office employee leaves, productivity will be affected, and revenues are likely to be lower. If s/he is a front office employee, the percentage of receivables collected is likely to decrease. Additionally, employee turnover generally reduces service quality and has a negative impact on patient satisfaction. While poor service may not have an immediate financial impact, it will affect a practice's long-term growth and reputation.

If an employee is competent and liked by patients, letting him or her go simply to avoid increasing his/her pay, or to find a "cheaper" replacement, is a poor decision. The replacement process is aggravating, and the doctor is unlikely to actually save money. The costs of losing a competent employee are difficult to quantify, but the less efficient the existing medical and business processes employed by the practice, the greater the costs will be. The reason for this is that the productivity level of an inefficient process is highly dependent on specific, key people. I have seen some practices where the loss of one person has virtually halted an entire billing process and/or significantly reduced the doctor's productivity and the amount of time s/he has available for providing higher margin services.

One way of expressing the cost of staff turnover in a medical practice (in addition to administrative costs paid) is in terms of a range of percentages. For example: this action might result in a 5 percent reduction in productivity, or a 5 percent decline in the collection ratio, depending on which employee is leaving. The net effect of either of these alternatives is a 5 percent reduction in total revenue. For a practice in which a key employee who is cross-trained and works in both the front and back offices leaves, both the productivity and the collections are likely to be affected. In such a case, the potential of reducing total revenue is as great as 10 percent. For a practice with a 65 percent overhead, this would produce a greater than 20 percent drop in profit! Doctors with higher overheads would see even more dramatic declines in their profit.

Efficient business and medical processes improve productivity; they also help reduce turnover. This is because efficient processes are more streamlined and better designed for achieving positive results, and they enable employees to take on more responsibility and diversify their jobs. Staff can become involved in multiple processes and are able to cross-train. For most people, performing a variety of tasks and taking on increased responsibility for those tasks increases their level of job satisfaction; this not only makes work more productive, but also more interesting. Streamlined processes also lessen the impact created by unavoidable turnover. It is easier to train a new employee in processes that "make sense," and when staff members have been cross-trained, more of them will be capable of helping to train new employees.

Since satisfaction with one's job and with one's salary are both critical issues to retaining good employees, an ideal strategy for reducing turnover is to focus on improving efficiency and productivity, both of which lead to these ends. The lower employee turnover rate that results will serve to increase a practice's productivity and profitability even further. As a result of this focus, staff will be more satisfied, the work environment will be improved, and the practice will enjoy higher profits.

Don't Lay Off Employees Just to Save Money

Companies often elect to cut overhead as a way of boosting profit. This is a strategy that is used in both good times and bad. For most companies, however, cutting overhead means cutting jobs and laying off employees, and results of this type of "cost cutting" can be positive or negative, depending on the company's approach. There is a well-known business axiom that states, "You cannot cut your way into prosperity." This is certainly true when cost cutting is the primary strategical focus for increasing profit. Know, however, that cost cutting can be effective as part of a more all-encompassing strategy.

The February 11, 2002, issue of *Business Week* cited four companies that cut jobs in 2001 in order to reduce costs. Sears cut 2,400 jobs, and Praxair cut 900. In the three to six months following announcement of these cuts, the shares of both companies rose 30%. In that same year, Palm cut 250 employees, and Providian Financial laid-off 550. Palm's shares dropped 50% on the following day, and Providian's dropped 90% over the following four-month period, with its shares never recovering. Clearly, investors differentiate between "good layoffs" and "bad." Within these four examples lies a lesson for doctors regarding how best to approach cost cutting in their practices.

Staff salaries typically account for 30% to 50% of a medical practice's overhead. This makes salaries an obvious target when attempting to reduce expenses. One of the most important principles that I learned from economics courses, however, is that an employee should never be eliminated without first eliminating the activities performed by that employee. Warren Buffet once said, "There is a right size staff for every business," and during the 1990-1991 recession, reducing staff size was instrumental in helping the economy get back on track and end the recession. These "cutbacks" worked only because businesses were able to create efficiencies through elimination of activities and, thereby, boost productivity concurrent with the layoffs. These changes enabled the employees remaining to accomplish more, with less.

This same strategy can work in many medical practices. It has been my experience that at least half of the activities performed in a busy medical practice are unnecessary and, thus, can be eliminated. The end result is that costs are lowered and quality is improved. As wasted activities and unnecessary interruptions are eliminated, there may be opportunity for reducing staff. An alternative possibility is that this will free up time for more productive use by the existing staff. Eliminating unnecessary activities through the use of more efficient processes and applying technology in more productive ways will result in lower overhead and in greater productivity, and this will translate into growth. Restructuring can often accomplish both of these goals.

In the *Business Week* example cited above, the author concluded that, "Wall Street punishes those who cut jobs solely to reduce costs but rewards those whose layoffs are part of a strategic plan." The layoffs at Sears were part of a restructuring plan that included the closure of 89 stores. Praxair redeployed its savings from reduced overhead by investing in new plants during the economic slowdown. For both companies, the layoffs were only part of larger strategic plans. Providian was the fifth largest credit card company and had grown by focusing on high-risk business. When the economy "went south," layoffs did nothing to address the flaws in the underlying business model. For Sears, the layoffs were part of an overall strategy; whereas, for Providian, layoffs *were* the strategy.

Eliminating unnecessary activities is an effective strategy in both good times and bad. A recession simply provides the excuse to do what should have been done all along. No matter how essential every task might seem, the odds are that a substantial number of those performed in any business are superfluous and can be eliminated. When enough tasks are eliminated through reengineering, entire staff positions often become redundant, leading to smaller, but more effective, staffs. If the savings resulting from these reductions are reinvested in areas that lead to further growth – even better! There are many opportunities of this type available in medicine. You can begin today by questioning the value that each task you and your staff perform contributes to your end results.

Determine Your Optimum Number of Employees

One of the largest overhead costs incurred by a medical practice is that of staff salaries. Physicians attempting to control this expense, without sacrificing quality, should work towards achieving *optimum staffing ratios.* It turns out that achieving this goal is easier said than done. How do we determine the ideal full-time employees to doctor ratio (FTE/Dr)? Doctors looking to their peers in hopes of finding useful benchmarks will find a wide variation in this ratio – even amongst doctors in the same specialty who have practices of comparable size. The variation in staffing ratios for medical practices is extreme, ranging from one FTE/Dr to as many as ten. In spite of this extreme range, one thing all practices have in common is that when you ask staff members to name the biggest problem facing their practices, most will respond with, "Understaffing" – regardless of how large their ratios are. Doctors will be unable to change this perception until they better understand how to utilize efficiently. One thing is clear: staffing ratios do have an impact on both productivity and costs – with the optimum ratio defined as that which achieves the highest level of productivity at the lowest cost.

Staffing ratios vary from practice to practice because of many factors: differences in patient volumes, levels of productivity, levels of efficiency, and each practice's complexity. To gain a better understanding of how difficult it is to determine optimum staff size, let us start with the simplest model – a practice with one doctor, one nurse, and three treatment rooms. The FTE/Dr ratio for this practice is one, as is typical in the high tech, "micro-practice" model. In this model, the doctor and one staff person divide duties, both doing whatever tasks need to be done to treat all the patients and complete all the paperwork.

What happens when we go from this simple, one doctor, one staff, three-treatment-room model to a practice with three doctors and nine treatment rooms? Carrying this simple model forward and maintaining its FTE/Dr ratio of one, we would have a staff size of three; however, what often happens instead is very different. As a practice grows to this size, staff size often triples to nine, increasing the FTE/Dr ratio to three. It now takes nine staff to accomplish what three once did. In general, the FTE/Dr ratio tends to increase as the size of a group increases – often exponentially. Additional staff *can* be utilized to increase productivity; however, in most cases, they only become "necessary" for handling the increased complexity and magnified inefficiencies brought about by a growing practice. Most often, the cost of the salaries for the "extra" six staff in our three-doctor practice example does not achieve its equivalent in benefits. In fact, because of inefficiencies, each staff person added beyond the optimum number generally provides only marginal return for his/her additional cost – often as little as 15% of this cost. This helps to explain why hiring additional staff can leave a practice with less profit and still feeling understaffed!

A study conducted by Toyota determined that when using traditional, dependent series processes, only this marginal benefit of 15% is gained from each additional employee hired. The researchers determined that at any given time, 85% of workers weren't performing actual "work". In reality, however, only 5% of the employees were actually "not working". Of the remaining 80%, 25% were performing unnecessary tasks, 30% were "waiting for something", and 25% were working inefficiently – effectively accomplishing the same as "not working". These "idle times" were created by bottlenecks, variation, waste, and a need for information that required interrupting other employees.

When staff size is optimized and FTE/Dr ratios lowered, a practice attains more than 15% benefit from added staff. To achieve this in our practices, we must first understand why the benefit achieved can drop so dramatically as staff size increases. The basic difficulty is that, within any practice, the volume and urgency of tasks fluctuate from minute to minute, hour to hour, and day to day. At one moment, the phone is quiet, and at another, it is "ringing off the hook." In the first instance, no staff members are required; yet, the second might require three people to handle the rush. The same holds true with every task within a practice – checking patients in or out, calling to verify insurance eligibility, entering demographic and billing data into a computer, providing patients with information, responding to patient questions, filing or retrieving medical records, opening and distributing mail, escorting patients to treatment rooms, quoting fees, or making return appointments. In spite of the fact that any staff person *should* be able to perform these duties when work is backed up, they often *cannot* (even when their own "assigned" tasks are "quiet" at the time) – usually because these staff members have not been cross-trained, or because processes are inefficient, office policies outdated, or job descriptions limited. At busy times, this leads to a feeling that staff size is suboptimal, even in a practice that maintains a high FTE/Dr ratio.

As a second example, assume that an office has two doctors and six staff members. How might this practice deal effectively with the "feast or famine" nature of the various tasks that fluctuate, seemingly randomly, at any given moment? Traditionally, the "fix" for busy times has been "simple" – add more staff! Observing the workflow in such an office, we would often see that half the staff is idle at any given point in time; yet, at others, six are not enough. It is likely that this practice will eventually increase its staff because there will be times throughout each day when the "perception" of being understaffed is "real"; yet, as staff are added, even greater numbers of them will be idle during slow times, and at peak times, any new staff hired will provide only marginal benefit. As a practice hires more and more personnel, the end result is often a staffing level that is too high when the office is slow and too low when the office is busiest – the proverbial "lose-lose" outcome. What tends to prevent a practice from increasing its staff size indefinitely is that it eventually reaches the point at which it can no longer afford to hire any more and, instead, continues on with backlogs and staff complaints about needing more help.

An alternative to constantly hiring more personnel is to focus on redesigning processes and workflows so that current staff members are able to utilize their time more efficiently and effectively. It is fact that even during busy periods, staff can be idle more than 50% of the time – time spent "waiting for something," looking for information (often interrupting another employee to obtain that information), or performing duties which could be eliminated (such as filing charts or entering charges from paper charge slips). When applied effectively, today's technology enables a practice to utilize this wasted time efficiently and avoid some of it altogether. This is possible because technology can be located anywhere in the practice, saving time through the elimination of geographic barriers, and because multiple duties can now be performed in parallel from any location in the office, enabling any temporarily idled employee, anywhere in the office, to not just answer the phone for the purpose of transferring the call elsewhere, but to complete any necessary "transaction" – such as responding to a patient question or scheduling an appointment. This use of previously wasted time greatly lessens the need for adding more staff.

The goal in the above example is for this staff of six to be capable of functioning during busy times as though it were a staff of nine. This can be made possible through cross-training and implementation of effective technology. This would not only save unnecessary additional expense, but it is likely that, should the practice feel a need to hire more staff, the purpose would be for increasing productivity rather than for reducing backlogs – a *proactive* as opposed to a *reactive* response.

Getting the Most from Your Employees

At a point when I felt I had become pretty good at reading people, an eye opening experience taught me that I still had a long way to go. The incident involved a staff member whom I felt was significantly underperforming. I told her that I wanted to meet with her after work to discuss her future with the practice, and she replied that this was quite a coincidence since she was planning to ask me for a meeting regarding this same issue. It so happened that, while I wanted to explain what she needed to do in order to keep her job, she had intended to meet for the purpose of asking for a raise, leaving me to wonder how our perceptions could be so different. It became clear that I was not as good at reading people as I had thought, and I realized that such "gaps" in perception between me and my staff had the potential of constraining the continued improvement of my practice.

A few years ago, I came across a study that helped to explain this situation. I was reviewing data from a survey conducted for *BusinessWeek* by Beta Research Corporation in June, 2007, and was amazed at the typical response from employees across a wide range of fields to the question, "Are you one of the top 10% of performers in your company?" Overall, 90% of the respondents answered, "Yes." Breaking this statistic down even further, 83% of the respondents who worked in large companies (ones with more than 1,000 employees) and 96% from smaller companies (with fewer than 50 employees) responded, "Yes". Although we know that a gap exists between perception and reality, this is a pretty wide gap! We can examine here how recognizing this enigma might help us in managing our practices.

We have all heard the expression that "perception is reality." If we believe this and are dealing with someone who isn't really perceiving the reality of a situation, we typically focus on changing that person's perception. There are times, however, when we should be employing the opposite strategy. For example, we actually do want our staff to perform in the top 10% – to achieve their perception of reality. We want to change reality to match our "audience's" perception of it. This is the approach we need to take with our office staff, 96% of whom, according to this *Business Week* survey, perceive themselves as being in the top 10% of performers.

BusinessWeek's survey tells us it is likely that most people we deal with, both in business and social settings, on a daily basis – including the doctors we know – believe they are in the top ten percent of their professions. How do we turn such "overly optimistic" perceptions into reality? There is probably no correct answer to this question; however, just knowing that this "performance/perception gap" exists is valuable information. The fact that our staff, typically, are overly optimistic regarding their abilities and contributions to the success of our practices is certainly something we need to consider when managing staff related issues, especially when we are dealing with those whom we feel are under-performing. As we seek ways to help them improve performance, we must be aware of the fact that we are walking a fine line between improving the situation and undermining it by reducing staff confidence and self-esteem.

Ideally, we all share the long-term goal of increasing the quality and performance of our medical practices. Regardless of how well we might be performing today, we must focus on continuous improvement in order to move our practices from good to great. I feel that this "Going from Good to Great" concept (as described by Jim Collins in his book of the same title) offers an answer to the question, "How do I motivate employees without undermining their confidence and self esteem?" Key factors in going from good to great are the support and expertise of the people who will help us along the way. We can effectively deal with (and motivate) our employees who already believe they are in the top ten percent of performers by letting them know that we recognize how "good" they already are. Following this acknowledgment, our discussions can move forward, focusing on improvement – on how they and the practice can move forward, from "good" to "great."

We encounter differences in individual perceptions of reality in most situations. Sometimes these differences can be quite wide, potentially putting those who do not understand the extent of this gap at a disadvantage. Simple awareness of this discrepancy can change how we interact with people in all situations, resulting in better outcomes from our interactions and a continuous, positive impact on both our business and personal lives.

Employee Performance Reviews Don't Need to Be Painful

Human resource consultants recommend that employees receive job performance reviews at least once a year. As essential as these reviews can be for the growth and wellbeing of employees, many doctors are uncomfortable with this process. As a result, they perform reviews infrequently, if at all. When one is performed, the process is often prompted by the need to document a specific employee's poor performance. Rather than using the review as a tool for improving employee performance, this information is used to avoid litigation when terminating someone. I argue that the avoidance of regular performance reviews might actually contribute to poor performance. Since employee turnover is costly and upbeat attitudes can improve both morale and productivity for the entire practice, wouldn't it be better to conduct performance reviews proactively with the intent of improving employee performance and avoiding turnover?

Doctors dislike performance reviews because they can become confrontational, often serving as "gripe sessions." This is unproductive and accomplishes nothing for the practice or the employee. Human resource consultants often suggest detailed reviews. These are often too complicated and mechanized, thereby reducing the opportunity for outcomes that will raise employee morale and motivate them to improve performance.

What type of reviews, then, should be conducted? Performance reviews typically follow an employee's job description. Even if the description is not in writing, the doctor should have an idea of what the employee's duties are so that s/he has a basis for formulating questions that call for the employee's ideas and input. The review, however, should not simply follow the job description in a "mechanized" manner. This does not offer the opportunity to broaden the discussion and include what the duties might, or should, include.

An effective review requires an interactive discussion and an open agenda, one that could possibly lead to the identification of problems for which the employee might suggest solutions. This enables employee growth, expands his/her role in and value to the practice, and increases job satisfaction. Since job satisfaction is the most important factor affecting an employee's attitude (and, hence, level of performance and value to the practice), an employee review should delve into areas that specifically include issues most important to that employee.

A successful review results in an employee who is motivated and excited to continue in his/her job. If the employee's job satisfaction needs are unmet, it is less likely that s/he will be motivated to focus on your needs. A 2010 survey conducted by the Society for Human Resource Management found the top seven areas most important to an employee's job satisfaction to be:

1. Job security	63%
2. Benefits	60%
3. Opportunity to use skills and abilities	56%
4. The organization's financial stability	54%
5. The work itself	54%
6. Salaries	53%
7. Recognition of the employee's job performance	48%

Job security is the number one concern for most people, and because of this, if you value an employee, you should make sure that s/he feels secure in his/her job and knows that you value his/her contribution to your practice. Many doctors are surprised that salary ranks number six on this list – behind benefits, which are in second place. Since benefits are valued so highly, when giving an

employee a raise, it might make sense to ask if s/he would prefer this raise to be in the form of a non-taxable benefit.
There are numerous ways for employees to expand their skills and abilities. Effective tools for accomplishing this are cross-training and empowerment – both of which contribute to higher productivity and lower costs. Learning new skills not only increases an employee's value, it opens the opportunity for lateral movement within the practice and creates greater job satisfaction. Increasing employee skills and abilities empowers staff and prevents them from feeling "stuck" and becoming bored, performing the same tasks year after year.

There is no single ideal way to conduct a performance review, but it is clear that an important opportunity is missed when reviews are avoided altogether. I suggest that when conducting a review, you find a way to include the above-listed, top-seven employee concerns associated with job satisfaction in your discussion. These can be added to the usual discussion of "routine" duties and will secure better outcomes from your formal reviews.

Invest in Your Staff

Teamwork is critical to getting things done in a medical practice. Building teamwork was one of the many things that John Wooden, the legendary former coach of the UCLA men's basketball team, was very good at. His philosophy of teamwork was based on an approach of on-going learning. Coach Wooden once said, "If I am through learning, I am through." He went on to say, "No matter how fine a person is at anything, he can always improve. No one ever reaches maximum potential." Wooden had some very talented players throughout his career, but he knew that raw talent alone wouldn't win championships. It fascinated me to watch coach Wooden's players improve continuously throughout their time at UCLA. All of us can approach our practices with this same attitude. The fact that we, our staff, and our practices can all continue to improve throughout our entire careers is an exciting prospect.

Studies have shown that fewer than 25% of improvement projects initiated in any type of business actually achieve positive outcomes. This percentage is so low because, in addition to knowing *how* to perform the tasks necessary for completion of a project, participants also need to understand *why* the tasks they perform are necessary. This is the reason I feel that, if a project is going to "work," it is important not only to train staff to perform their specific tasks, but also to explain why you believe those tasks are necessary to the project as a "whole." The more your staff understands the purpose for what they are doing, the more adept they will become at solving problems themselves and suggesting better ways of doing things.

Continuing education is essential for both doctors and staff; it is here that everyone can learn both the "how" and the "why" of practice improvement projects. Doctors clearly recognize the value of increasing their own skills and knowledge through regular participation in continuing education programs. Through this process, they learn from experts in the field and have the opportunity to exchange ideas with peers attending the same lectures and workshops. Physicians often return from these meetings feeling reenergized and excited to return to their practices; yet, interestingly, while they recognize this value for themselves, many don't seem to recognize the value that their staffs can obtain from attending the same type of programs.

To highlight the impact that recognizing this value might have on your practice, consider that an assistant spends, on average, twice the time the doctor does with patients – answering questions and explaining what the doctor has just told them. In this age of instant information on the web, the assistant must have the most up-to-date information regarding his/her field. In many cases, patients have already done their homework on the latest treatments, techniques, and procedures – as well as products – and assistants need to be ahead of them. The best way for this to happen is for staff to stay current by keeping up through educational programs.

Is employee training worth the investment? Consider the following benefits to be gained from continuing education and training for your staff:

1. Increased job satisfaction and morale amongst staff members
2. Increased employee motivation

3. Increased efficiencies in processes – resulting in financial gain
4. Increased acceptance by employees of new methods and technologies
5. Increased innovation in strategies and products offered
6. Reduced employee turnover – resulting in reduced recruiting and training costs
7. An enhanced office image
8. Improved risk management
9. Anticipation of potential office issues – with the advantage of catching problems before they escalate
10. Enhanced patient satisfaction and loyalty

Many doctors recognize that they need staff members who can turn on a dime, individuals who have the capability of doing today what they could not do last year. To achieve this, staff members need continuous training – not just training regarding a new product, skill, or software program, but also training that is designed to improve overall performance. Today's medical world is expanding quickly, and to keep up-to-date, a staff must be learning continuously. Training should involve specific products, procedures, process information, and techniques for building relationships with both peers and patients. Training develops employee motivation and loyalty, which in turn, lead to higher productivity on the job. It is important to ask yourself, "What will happen if I don't continue to train my staff?"

Pay Your Receptionist Fairly

The Professional Association of Health Care Office Management (PAHCOM) regularly conducts surveys, gathering a variety of statistical information about its members. One finding of its 2002 annual survey caught my attention – the response to the question, "What medical staff position is most difficult to fill with qualified people?" *Table 5.1* illustrates the top four responses to this question, showing that "receptionist" is considered the most difficult position to fill with a qualified person, and this response led "nursing staff," the second place response, by a wide margin.

Table 5.1: Response to the question, "What staff position is most difficult to fill?"

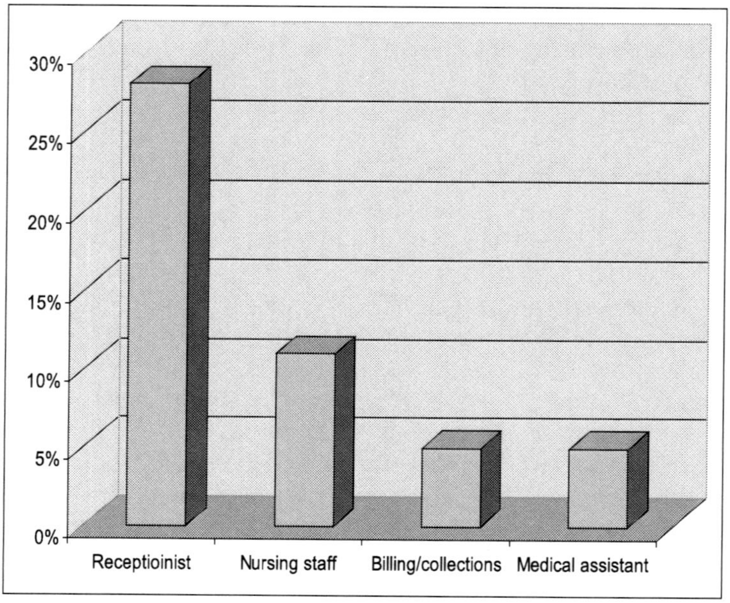

National averages for staff salaries at the time of PAHCOM's queries are shown in *Table 5.2*. It should be no surprise that the position for which medical practices feel it is most difficult to find qualified personnel also happens to be at the bottom of the pay scale. The only position with an average salary lower than that of the receptionist is the filing clerk, a position which, when compared to that of receptionist, requires little to no qualifications, interpersonal skills, or experience.

Many physicians mistakenly place low value on the position of receptionist, seeing it as requiring few qualifications and little experience. In fact, they seem to feel that the primary qualification for the job is, "A person who is willing to work for very little." I am not sure how this misperception has come about, but my feeling is that it is based on the assumption that, by age eighteen, everyone should know how to "answer a phone and be nice to people." Following a medical receptionist through a "typical" day makes it obvious that the position entails much more than this.

Table 5.2: 2002 Average staff salaries, nationally

Position	National Average
Office manager	$50,687
Assistant office manager	$34,665
Collections clerk	$27,675
Billing clerk	$26,752
Bookkeeper	$26,371
Insurance clerk	$25,414
Transcriber	$25,242
Data entry clerk	$23,488
Receptionist	$22,408
Filing clerk	$18,431

The duties of a receptionist vary widely for each practice, but they always involve greeting patients as they arrive at the front desk. In addition, s/he might check patients in, gather demographic and insurance information, enter this information into a computer, answer the phone, make appointments, pull charts, collect co-pays, answer questions, deliver messages, and even cover for other staff members when they are unavailable. With all of these responsibilities, "just" answering the phone or "being nice to everyone" is not always easy – especially during peak periods.

Roger Landers, PAHCOM'S business manager and editor of its newsletter, would like to see higher salaries for receptionists because, as he writes, "It's such a stressful job and has a high burnout rate." Doctors need to recognize that this is actually a key position with high visibility and a great deal of responsibility. The effective performance of a receptionist's daily responsibilities (which are necessary for the efficient flow of patients and often occur simultaneously), impact two highly valued processes within the practice – marketing and operations – both of which, in turn, impact reimbursement.

Courtesy and efficiency of staff are among the most significant measures of patient satisfaction, and the first contact patients have with a practice is with the receptionist. Consider the amount of money that many doctors spend on various types of marketing and advertising to attract new patients. They could achieve a better return on this investment by using more of these dollars to find and retain good receptionists. This staff member plays a significant role in the practice's cash flow and collection ratio because s/he is located at the front end of the reimbursement process. Mistakes made or incorrect/incomplete information obtained when a patient first arrives, can result in uncollected co-pays, underpaid third party claims, or claim rejections. I outlined earlier why finding and fixing these initial mistakes at a later time is difficult and costly. It is important that they be prevented at the beginning of the process. Mistakes, errors, and delays occur far more frequently at peak periods, when the phone is "ringing off the hook," multiple patients are checking in or out, the waiting room is full, and the doctor is running behind. This is when an experienced, competent receptionist offers a practice significant value. This is not a job for the fainthearted, and it is definitely not a position to be filled by the lowest paid or least skilled member of the team.

Call Centers Can Reduce the Burden on Your Receptionist

One strategic outsourcing opportunity commonly used in industry is the routing of incoming calls to a call center. These centers can be located anywhere in the world and can be used to handle such things as customer service, sales orders, and appointment scheduling. Many doctors consider the use of a call center for their practices; unfortunately, when making the decision of whether or not to use one, they primarily focus on cost savings, rather than on strategic benefits that might be gained from their use. If the reason for utilizing a call center is simply to have someone answer the phone, putting it into service is not a strategic move because cost reduction is the only consideration; however, a call center can provide more than simply "a person who answers the phone."

If you ever visit a busy practice during a "peak period" and it is one that uses a call center effectively, you will immediately be struck by how calm the front office appears to be. Patient satisfaction is high because the staff feels less rushed, patients are recognized and greeted courteously as they arrive, and there are no long lines waiting to be checked-in or out. From a strategic standpoint, an effective call center that generates high levels of patient satisfaction positions a practice for growth. It also produces "non-visible" benefits, including a higher collection ratio and greater practice profitability.

Let us take a look at where call centers fit into the workflow of a practice to see what types of opportunities can be captured through their use. Typically, outside calls coming to an office are answered directly at the front desk. Depending on the size of the practice, these calls are answered by a designated receptionist or a multi-tasking front office person who is responsible for a myriad of tasks, including: greeting patients, checking them in, gathering demographic and insurance information, entering that information into a computer, assembling medical records, collecting co-pays, making return appointments, and checking patients out.

In a busy practice, an incoming call is almost always treated as an interruption because the person answering the call is required to stop whatever s/he is doing in order to respond. This person is often in the process of assisting a patient who is standing in front of him/her. The receptionist feels rushed, the in-office patient feels ignored, and if the number of phone calls and the patient flow are all exceeding capacity at the same time, call-in patients are put on hold, lines begin to form at check-in and check-out points, the staff becomes even more rushed, courtesy is "tested," and the number of data entry errors, omissions, and delays increases – all factors eventually leading to a lower collection ratio. A call center can change this by diverting incoming calls away from this "bottle-necked" front desk location to a dedicated "answerer" who has the time and expertise to patiently handle them.

If you decide to use a call center, it is imperative that you work with the optimal software. Because an examination of workflow shows us that a call center serves as the first step of both the billing and the new patient appointment scheduling processes, the ideal is for the call center and the practice to use the same software.

Consider an environment in which, when a new patient calls in, the person answering has ample time to spend on the phone with the patient, make an optimal appointment, accurately enter all demographic and insurance information directly into the practice's database, and answer all the patient's questions. When efficient software and an effective call center are in place, the average time required to accomplish all of this is less than three minutes. This creates "extra" time for in-office employees to make follow-up calls (such as those required to verify eligibility, or obtain prior authorizations) and locate previous lab tests, x-rays, or medical records that might be needed at the time of treatment.

A reduction in data entry errors (created through the use of an "unhurried" staff) also dramatically increases the collection ratio, and having a patient's information in place in the database before s/he arrives at the practice expedites the check-in process. Imagine a patient who arrives at the front desk with all demographic and insurance information already uploaded into the system. Because all "preliminary" work has been completed, the person checking the patient in has the time to re-check the computer's insurance information against the patient's insurance card. This process, along with the practice software, helps to identify errors, collect co-pays, and notify the back office "electronically" when the patient has arrived and is ready to be brought back to a treatment room. Fully integrated software enables an unhurried, accurate, efficient, initial contact between a patient and the practice.

A call center can help you attain these results whether that center is located in-house or elsewhere. One might be developed through the collaborative efforts of a number of independent doctors who come together to outsource this function to a shared staff located at a separate facility, or it might be individually outsourced to an independent company located anywhere in the world. Regardless of where the call center is located, in order to enable optimal scheduling, the most strategically effective center will utilize appointment software that is embedded with the office's scheduling rules. With the use of effective software, embedded with your rules, a call center can help you to eliminate some of the most common and recurrent problems experienced by the majority of medical practices.

Is it a Bad Idea to Hire Family Members?

A question that doctors frequently ask practice management "experts" is whether or not it is wise to hire family members to work in their medical practices. There are good arguments on both sides of this issue, but many base their arguments on emotion and fear rather than on logic and real world evidence. If you are considering this option, you want to be certain that your judgment is based on the latter. Do not automatically rule out this possibility, especially if you are doing so based on the mis-belief that this is destined to be a bad idea.

Over a decade ago, I compared the practice of family members working in medical offices to successful "mom and pop" businesses in which one or more of the "employees" were family members. I pointed out that these businesses tend to be highly efficient and effective because employed family members are typically committed, empowered, and cross-trained. All of these factors tend to expand productivity and reduce overhead. During my first decade in practice, I noted that the majority of respected practice management speakers who, at the time were practitioners themselves, typically employed their spouses. Upon observation of these practices, it became clear that the spouses working in these offices were trained to perform any and all functions and were empowered to make decisions. For me, this raised the question of, "Why not cross-train and empower all employees?" – essentially, treat all staff as "family members."

The researchers of a "Special Report" published in the November 10, 2003, issue of *BusinessWeek* found that one-third of S&P 500 companies had founding families involved in management. More importantly, those companies with family members involved in the business were found to be amongst the best performers. These "family businesses" included companies such as Wrigley, Walgreens, Alberto-Culver, and Wal-Mart. The researchers of this article attributed the successful performance of these companies to the following five factors: 1) born to lead, 2) quick decisions, 3) breeding loyalty, 4) investing in growth, and 5) no absentee landlords.

Born to lead

Imagine the advantage of growing up in a family that is running a successful business. Consider the positive attitudes, the mentoring environment, and the advice available from elders. Family members are "groomed" for company leadership from the start.

Similarly, this type of environment is created in families where one of the members has built a successful medical practice.

Quick decisions

The article notes that family corporations run by a few tight-knit family members can "move" faster than the typical corporate bureaucracy. This flexibility offers one of the biggest advantages that "small" private practices have when competing with larger groups and is especially important when it comes to capturing new opportunities.

Breeding loyalty

Loyalty reduces turnover and increases productivity. In families, loyalty is "built in." Most doctors understand the value of a loyal employee and will go to great lengths to retain one in their practices. Family employees are loyal to the business, and family run businesses are more likely to treat non-family employees as if they were family members too. They tend to provide their employees with family type benefits such as day care, profit-sharing, and resistance to layoffs during downturns.

Investing in Growth

Companies that are family-run tend to reinvest heavily in their businesses. The writers of this *BusinesWeek* article stated that the average family-run business in the S&P 500 reinvested $79 million more for research, development, and growth than the average non-family-run business. It is easy to understand how ownership fosters an environment in which cash is reinvested in growing the business and where there is resistance to taking money out of the business for spending elsewhere.

No absentee landlords

A family member who has both a personal and financial stake in a business has a greater incentive to hold management accountable.

Years of growing up in a business also gives him/her detailed knowledge of that business, making it easier to evaluate management.

An important "take home point" from this brief analysis is that advantages similar to those found in successful family run businesses can be attained in private medical practices by actually hiring family members or simply by treating all employees as family members. Employing trust, empowerment and cross-training and offering valued social and financial benefits create loyalty, leadership, and a sense of ownership in all employees – whether they are actually family or not. As with any practice decision, the one of whether or not to employ a family member should be based on logic, facts, and what will be best for the practice. If "mom and pop" businesses make sense for many successful Fortune 500 companies, who are we to rule out this option for our practices?

Spend Less Time Fixing Blame, and More Time Fixing Inefficient Processes

When participating in management seminars, I am often asked if there is a new technique, a "pearl," that can be implemented in a practice "overnight," one which might measurably increase the performance of that practice. In reality, most changes that are capable of improving medical practice performance require significant effort and rarely can be fully implemented in a day, a week, or even a month; however, there is a management *approach* that can be implemented virtually overnight which, when employed, helps to prevent the same problems from occurring over and over again.

Problem solving skills are a prerequisite to running a successful business, and the business of medicine is no exception. Examining how we, as doctors, spend our days brings us to the realization that the majority of our time is spent solving problems. As doctors, we are trained to solve clinical problems, but because our practices are businesses, we must also be capable of solving business problems.

How do we approach clinical problem solving? We begin with a history, perform an examination, order tests, and take X-rays. We then evaluate this information in light of our experience, with the goal of identifying the underlying cause of a patient's problems so that we can "cure" him/her. This cure will require that 1) we prescribe a treatment plan and 2) the patient understand the reasons for our recommendations so that we can achieve maximum compliance. If we do our job well, we not only eliminate our patient's symptoms, but we also fix the underlying causes of those symptoms so that they do not return. While we recognize this as the best approach to patient care, many of us do not employ the same, successful approach for solving our business problems.

Many managers do not search for underlying causes when problems occur. Instead, they search for someone to blame. Focus turns to fixing blame rather that fixing problems. Most managers are unaware that they do this, which results in a continuation, or worsening, of existing problems. A change in this approach can lead to major improvement in business performance. Dr. W. Edwards Deming, the guru of efficient, high quality manufacturing processes, estimates that, "Most troubles and most possibilities for improvement add up to proportions something like 94 percent that belong to the system." The same is true for errors (both medical and business) that occur in our practices. Doctors do not prevent medical errors by being smarter; they prevent them through the employment of smarter processes, ones that are efficient, track tasks, and have built-in controls. In a medical practice, the "system" referred to by Deming as being responsible for "most troubles" is the collection of tasks that make up our business processes, the processes that deliver services to patients, staff, and third parties.

When we blame an employee for something that has "gone wrong" in our practices, 94% of the time, the "fault" is not the staff's. Instead, responsibility actually lies in our business and management processes, ones that we, and not the employees, have designed and put in place. Blaming an employee never fixes an underlying cause; this only creates an environment in which employees attempt to hide their errors for fear of being reprimanded. Accused employees become afraid to experiment or suggest changes that might actually fix a "system," and this allows the same, or similar, problems to persist. Since new problems will continue to arise, regardless of how competent a staff may be, a doctor who uses an approach focused on fixing blame will assure that his/her practice achieves continuous decline rather than continuous improvement.

We must accept the fact that we will always encounter problems in our practices. What we should not accept is for the same problems to recur over and over again. The value of our skill as managers is measured by how we approach and solve problems. Any time spent fixing blame is wasted and leads neither to real solutions nor to a motivated, productive staff. When a mistake occurs – such as when a chart or a test is missing, a patient arrives without an authorization, a co-pay is not collected, a charge slip is not marked, or a third party payment is delayed because of "missing information" – the emphasis should be placed on identifying *why* the mistake occurred rather than on *who* made the mistake. Once the cause has been identified, doctors and staff can work on finding and implementing a creative solution directed at that underlying cause. This will actually "fix" the problem because it prevents future recurrences.

Doctors who want to test the effectiveness of a "solution" can develop reports that track the occurrence of a specific type of mistake, measure its frequency, and provide objective feedback that will identify whether the instituted "solution" is actually reducing the frequency of the mistake's recurrence. The biggest payoff achieved from this approach is that it sets a continuous mechanism in motion whereby practice performance is constantly improved. Rather than focusing on putting out fires, everyone is seeking ways of preventing them. This leaves more time for reviewing reports and tackling strategic problems; performance improves continuously, and everyone's job becomes more productive and more satisfying.

When asked to what they attribute their success, most successful physicians unhesitatingly cite their staffs. For the majority of these doctors, staff salaries account for thirty to fifty percent of their practice overhead. Because this is such a significant investment, it is important that doctors find and hold on to the best staff members possible. Successful managers realize that even the best employees will make mistakes and that an environment of fixing blame will quickly result in the loss of talented ones. Fixing problems, however, generates a stimulating environment, one that leads to a sense of accomplishment. Imagine the level of productivity that can be achieved by talented staff members who tackle new problems with no fear of retribution for unsuccessful initial attempts.

At first glance, it would seem that switching from a "fixing blame" to a "fixing causes" approach would be something that could be implemented overnight. While this is certainly possible, the reality is that changing any habit can be extremely difficult, and for many, this is a habit. Habits are automatic – responses that we seldom even recognize we have. When a manager reacts by pointing a finger and fixing blame, the implied message is that this problem is not his/her fault and that s/he shares none of the responsibility for it. This makes no sense; it certainly does not help in solving problems. Accepting responsibility, however, moves the discussion away from fixing blame (where there are no good outcomes). We all recognize that, by definition, the person in charge is ultimately responsible for everything that happens, regardless of when, or by whom, a mistake is made. The doctor is the person in charge of a medical practice, and everything that happens, both good and bad, is ultimately his/her responsibility. Whenever a mistake or an oversight leads to a problem, a successful doctor/manager must take responsibility and motivate everyone to focus on the "fix" along with finding ways to prevent the same thing from recurring in the future. This is what leaders do. It puts staff at ease and secures their active assistance in finding and implementing solutions. Although it can be difficult to change a mindset, the sooner the focus of a practice is turned from fixing blame to fixing causes, the sooner that practice can capture a continuous flow of process improvement.

Chapter 6

Fix Your Scheduling Process

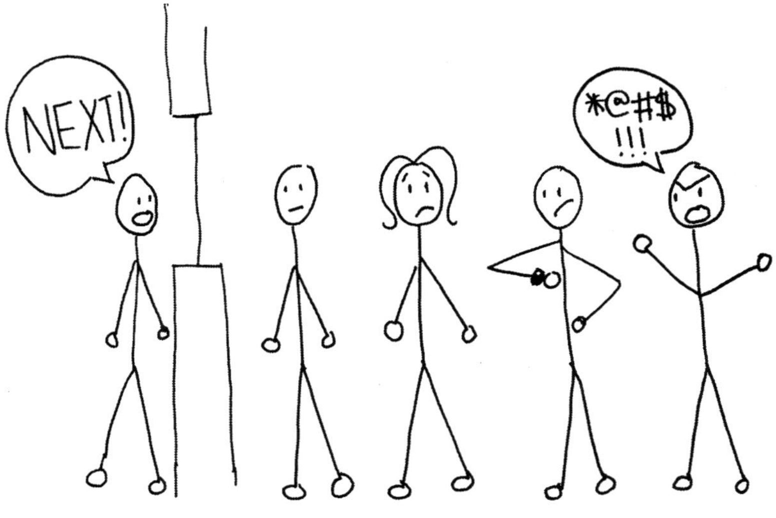

Why Proper Scheduling Is Important

Medical practices are classic examples of the "high fixed cost" economic model. In a medical business, the costs considered "fixed" are those unaffected by increases or decreases in patient volume – ones that remain constant. Included in these costs, which account for the majority of the overhead in a medical practice, are: rent, salaries, and malpractice insurance. In spite of the disadvantages of its high costs, there are ways of taking advantage of this model. When volume and/or fees of an efficiently run, high fixed cost business are increasing, a large percentage of the additional revenue produced is realized as profit because revenue increases disproportionately to costs. The problem with this model, however, is that the opposite occurs when volume and/or fees are decreasing – profit is reduced. The paradox is that today's doctors are practicing in an environment in which volume is increasing while fees are decreasing, pulling profit in opposite directions.

Efficiency has proven to be an effective means of addressing the costs and potential for lower quality associated with increased volume; however, it can be difficult to determine what it is that needs to be made efficient. When faced with a practice hurdle, it is helpful to study other industries that have high fixed costs similar to those of the medical practice. This exercise can provide insight into possible approaches for solving a variety of problems. Many industries have already faced environments with increasing volume and decreasing fees and found solutions for addressing the problems that result. While our solutions won't be exactly the same as the ones that "worked" for other industries, the underlying science used to identify causes and develop solutions for problems of similar origin will be the same.

Let us review an example in the shipping industry. When faced with low profits, the "conventional wisdom" of the industry told them that their ships needed to be made more efficient. New, faster and more fuel-efficient ships were developed; however, this did not seem to change the negative economics of the industry. It was not until experts "discovered" that the industry's low profit was actually a result of inefficiencies "in port" – when cargo was being loaded and unloaded – rather than inefficiency of the ships at sea. A ship in port generates costs while producing no income. Similarly, a medical practice produces no income each hour that it is idled (not seeing patients), but the fixed costs (rent, staff salaries, insurance, etc.) continue to mount whether patients are being seen or not. The shipping industry finally solved its principal revenue problem by focusing on the efficiency of its "in port" cargo turnover. The solution included the invention of roll-on, roll-off containers, which increased throughput and made the entire loading/unloading process faster, and thus, more efficient.

A parallel to the "in-port inefficiency" dilemma faced by the shipping industry can be found in our medical practices. This is the inefficiency present in the process of treatment room turnover, especially as a practice's patient volume approaches capacity. As patient volume increases and a practice adds doctors or merges with other practices, the treatment room turnover rate becomes a limiting factor to practice efficiency and growth. Slow treatment room turnover results in longer waits for patients and doctors who lose valuable treatment time as they wait for rooms to "open up" for patients. Physicians typically "solve" this problem by adding capacity – increasing the square footage of their offices and/or the number of staff – both solutions that push the already high fixed costs of their practice even higher and the profit percentages lower. Our shipping industry example shows us how a similar problem in another industry was solved. The same laws governing throughput are applicable to medical practices, and understanding them can provide us with more innovative and efficient ways of scheduling the use of our treatment rooms as well as physician and staff time.

Looking to the Skies for Answers

To gain some insight into solving this problem, let us look at the airline industry, which faces a similar problem. Running "on time" provides a marketing advantage for an airline, just as it does for a medical practice. While the airlines have made great strides in improving their "on time" performance, the fact that major airlines now fill most of their seats presents a familiar challenge – "loading and unloading." Planes can often sit idle at gates for long periods of time while arriving passengers unload and departing ones board. For marketing purposes, it is important that airlines be on time, and as it turns out, there are also reasons related to the high fixed costs of the industry that make it imperative that they develop efficient passenger "turnover" processes.

According to Andrew Miller, CEO of Centre for Asia Pacific Aviation, "Every extra minute a plane sits on the ground adds up to tens of millions of dollars." "Fixed costs" soar as airlines increase the amount of time they spend on the ground. Southwest estimates that if its boarding time were to increase by ten minutes per flight, just maintaining its current number of flights would require an additional forty planes (at a cost of $40 million each!). Even more costs would be incurred due to the need for additional pilots, flight attendants, fuel, and gate space for each of these new planes, with no offsetting financial benefit.

The airlines are a good illustration of how inefficiency in "loading and unloading" a location (in this case, the plane), impacts a business's costs and customer satisfaction. It is critical for physicians to understand that when their practices are inefficient in this same process (the utilization of time and space), it is proportionately as costly for them as it is for these other businesses. Adding capacity in the form of more office space and/or staff generates even more costs and should be considered only after first fixing efficiency problems that will persist and continue to create problems even if capacity is increased.

The airlines hired mathematicians, physicists, and engineers to help them improve their workflow issues. One thing these experts determined was that the conventional process of loading a plane "back to front" was not the most efficient. In fact, according to Dr. Eitan Bachmat, a physicist at Ben-Gurion University, "Boarding a plane back to front is slower than simply letting people file on at random." Currently, each airline is testing various boarding models (such as the window seats first, middle seats next, and aisle seats last) to determine which will, ultimately, prove to be most effective. The important thing to recognize here is that airlines are "experimenting" with alternatives and measuring the results, and this will eventually lead to finding better processes. Physicians, too, should be examining the processes that affect their treatment room turnover rate. They should begin "experimenting" with alternative processes in appointment scheduling and communication channels between the front and back offices, with the goal of optimizing utilization of both office space and personnel.

A medical practice has tools for creating more efficient room turnover, and these are: effective communication processes between the front desk and the "back" treatment areas, well-designed appointment books, and efficient scheduling processes that accommodate the variation that exists in the "average" appointment time slot. An effective communication process offers a way to alert the back office staff when patients arrive and to let them know when patients are ready to be brought back to treatment rooms. When a front office backlog begins to develop, creating delays that idle back office staff, those in the back office should be cross-trained so that they can communicate with the front office and assist them in their tasks, thus helping to eliminate these temporary backlogs.

An efficient scheduling process can help to reduce bottlenecks in patient flow. Most busy practices still use the same scheduling processes they did when their patient volumes were low, and they have kept the same appointment and workflow processes, even following the introduction of computerization. Most use an appointment book with all time slots of equal length, each representing an "average treatment time." A process that utilizes the advantages that can be captured through use of an effective computerized scheduling program can change all of this and revolutionize a practice's patient flow.

Scheduling and moving patients to treatment rooms can be compared to moving passengers on and off planes. Patients scheduled for five minutes can be thought of as window seat passengers, ones for fifteen minutes as those in middle seats, and ones scheduled for twenty minutes as passengers on the aisle. A new patient is the passenger who takes extra time to board because s/he needs assistance. Design of efficient workflow processes can prevent patients scheduled for twenty-five minutes from being brought back and seen in front of ones scheduled for only five. Purposeful scheduling with attention to workflow will result in more effective use of treatment rooms, create shorter patient wait times and, in turn, increase office capacity. What is most important in the design of practice workflow processes is that the steps in those processes be based on scientific principles and their results measured. This approach delivers the highest likelihood of success, and this is why the airlines utilized the expertise of mathematicians, physicists, and engineers to help solve their throughput problem.

Understanding and applying the science of workflow and throughput to the scheduling process is what enabled my practice to double its capacity and add more doctors to the group. We accomplished this without adding staff or space; we "simply" utilized a new workflow strategy that significantly lowered the overhead percentage and increased the profit margin. Most importantly, patient satisfaction also increased because of the quicker practice access and shorter patient wait times that resulted from our improved workflow processes.

Variation and Your Scheduling Process

Assume that a doctor who sees an average of twenty patients a day sets a goal of doubling that average volume to forty. Though the current average volume is twenty, we know that daily numbers vary. For example, in one sample week, the doctor might see one hundred patients: fifteen on Monday, twenty-five on Tuesday, ten on Wednesday, thirty on Thursday, and twenty on Friday. These one hundred patients average exactly twenty a day; however, the variation in volume throughout this week ranges from a low of ten to a high of thirty per day. For this practice to average twenty patients a day, it must have the capacity to see thirty on any given day. Because many physicians perform surgery or specialized services that eliminate office treatment time several half-days a week – and they take days off for meetings, seminars, vacations, and illness – in order to average twenty-patient days, practices must, on some days, be able to see even more than thirty.

For the sake of simplicity, assume that forty is the greatest number of patient visits this doctor must be capable of seeing in order to average twenty a day. This means that if the doctor wants to double average daily volume, s/he must be prepared on a given day to see double the peak volume of forty. While I personally know physicians who are capable of seeing this number of patients in one day, this is not easy, and an option would be to add a doctor and/or physician extender to the practice. This not only increases the possibility of doubling the average patient volume without adding to wait times, but it also reduces the peak volume needed, per doctor, to average forty patients a day and provide coverage of the practice during each doctor's surgery time and days off. In other words, operations are improved by a combination of increasing capacity and reducing the wide variation in the hourly and daily volume range necessary to achieve the average. Even when adding the appropriate personnel to help treat an increase in patient volume, this appointment variation problem must be effectively addressed to prevent "temporary" treatment room shortages throughout the day.

Variation not only constrains practice growth by creating the potential for overwhelming "peak" days, it also comes into play when considering the amount of time required for each individual patient visit. Appointment books are typically designed to allow fixed time slots for patient visits. Although the amount of time allotted, per visit, might represent the average length of a visit, actual visit times vary greatly.

Consider an appointment book constructed to allow an average of ten minutes for each visit. The hope is that, even though the time required for each visit will vary, forty visits will average out to be ten minutes each by the end of the day. For example, though one patient might require six minutes, and another fourteen, the average for the two visits will be ten. This variation from the norm can create bottlenecks. As we learned in earlier chapters, the "pluses and minuses" for the individual tasks in a dependent series process such as this do not average out; instead, the minuses accumulate, leading to back ups in patient flow that create patient waits which, at times, can be long.

Even when an appointment book is more sophisticated and breaks down office visits by type (such as new patient, consultation, follow-up, procedure, or post-op), there is still a wide range of time required for visits within each visit type. In most cases, appointment time slots allow the same amount of time for each category of visit, regardless of the patient's condition. Even though the length of time for a follow up visit may vary significantly, the appointment secretary books them all for an equal amount of time. Addressing this scheduling predicament can lead to efficient patient flow and increased productivity.

How can we avoid setting inappropriate length appointment times? Simple awareness of the fact that volume and time variation exists is the first step in reducing the impact of this problem. Understanding the potential effects of variation is critical for doctors who seek to increase volume without sacrificing patient satisfaction. Strategies designed to reduce variation can have a significant, positive impact on cost and quality, especially when volume is increasing. For this reason, doctors seeking practice growth should not only be developing marketing plans, they should also be developing operational plans to address the daily volume and time variation inherent in their patients' visits.

Decentralization Reduces Scheduling Variation Issues

In the early days of managed care, UCLA sought ways to decrease its costs. In the name of "efficiency," the hospital centralized appointment scheduling for all of its clinics. Rather than making return appointments from the clinics, patients were asked to call central scheduling. This may have reduced payroll costs, but more money was lost in revenue (in terms of physician productivity and patient satisfaction) than was saved in these costs. How is it possible for a receptionist working off site, with little or no clinical training, to schedule optimum appointments for every possible type of return visit? The resultant schedule was one which allocated too much time for some patients and too little for others, creating the proverbial lose-lose situation – longer waits for patients and less productivity from doctors.

In reality, no process works optimally when it is totally centralized. A hybrid generally works best – where some process tasks are centralized and others decentralized, with each being performed at its optimal location. Most practices employ a "centralized" form of scheduling in which a receptionist who is located at the front desk is the sole appointment maker. This person generally has the least clinical knowledge; and yet, s/he is responsible for appointing all patients – both those who call in by phone and those who schedule return visits when exiting the office.

Many call-in patients are new and require extra time for acquainting them with the practice and gathering their information. The appointments for these patients are generally of predictable length – allowing enough time for data entry, a complete history, exams, tests, and treatment. Exiting patients, on the other hand, are already "in the computer system," and appointing them requires no data entry. The amount of time they require for follow-up appointments does, however, vary widely – ranging from as little as five minutes to more than thirty. Unfortunately, regardless of the actual time required for each specific visit, when these patients are scheduled at the front desk, generally, they all are given appointments of "equal" length because the receptionist has little idea of the resources or amount of time necessary for treating specific conditions. When a receptionist double-books a time slot, it is just as likely that s/he will double-book two twenty minute patients in a fifteen minute slot as it is that s/he will put two five minute patients in that same slot. This is a universal problem that can be improved by decentralizing the process of *return visit* scheduling – entrusting this task to clinical staff or the doctor, team members who are better able to predict the amount of time optimal for each return visit.

Return visits can be made most effectively by clinical staff because they have thorough knowledge of each patient's condition, why s/he is returning, and as a result, how much time his/her particular visit will require. Even more specifically, they will know how much of the total appointed time will require the doctor's presence (this will be less than the amount of time needed by each patient for the treatment room), enabling them to optimize doctor, staff, and room time. An added bonus is the fact that exiting patients no longer have to interrupt the receptionist or wait in line, only to be given suboptimal appointments. The end result of decentralizing this portion of the scheduling process is a true win-win: patient waiting times are reduced, and the doctor is afforded more productive treatment time.

Decentralization of the rescheduling portion of the appointment process also affords the receptionist more time for greeting arriving patients, scheduling new patients, collecting patient co-pays and balances, and entering demographic and insurance information correctly (something which makes patient check-in/check-out more efficient and improves the billing process). On those occasions when clinical staff members are unavailable to make return appointments, the receptionist can perform this task as a secondary, rather than a primary, function.

Use a Large Appointment Book

The primary purpose of an appointment book is to help us plan each day effectively. The smaller the physical size of the "book," the more constrained planning becomes. It is surprising that some practices that have not yet transitioned to a computerized scheduling process continue to utilize limited, "week-at-a-glance," appointment books, which provide only one vertical column for each day of the week. While this may seem to work when first starting a practice, as patient volume grows, the receptionist has to write smaller and smaller to fit patients into the slots. Notes relevant to specific visits must be written in the margins or "squeezed" into the tiny time slots themselves. Little thought is given to the order in which patients arrive; rather, slots are filled randomly as patients call in.

When visiting one doctor's practice at a time prior to medical office computerization, I remember seeing a "fully booked" schedule that contained only two new patients, and they had been appointed back-to-back in the last two slots of the day. Rather than spacing these new patients apart so that the doctor would be allowed enough time to effectively evaluate their conditions, these appointments were "squeezed together" at the end of the day – determined by default – by the design of the appointment book. This just happened to be where their visits "physically" fit into the book itself.

Some practitioners who have implemented computerized appointment books tend to stay with their original designs, even as their practices change. In the past, the simplest "fix" for this variation dilemma was to design a book with large "slots" and multiple, vertical columns for each day, and while this is an improvement, an unlimited number of formats can be devised.

You can tailor one specifically to your needs. Just remember that, regardless of how you design your "book," it will be effective only if it provides sufficient space for planning. In the past, these "oversized" paper appointment books created a better mechanism for addressing the scheduling variation problem as practices became busier; however, because there was just one "book," it needed to be located at the front desk, with all return visits being made in a dependent series fashion by a receptionist. The advent of process computerization has changed all this.

Increase the Size of Your Fish Bowl

There is probably no greater constraint to practice growth than having an insufficient number of "slots" in the appointment book. If you ask a number of physicians, "How many patients do you see on a fully booked day?" you will receive widely varying responses. Some consider themselves to be "fully booked" at fifteen patients a day, while others are comfortable seeing thirty. If you were to ask these same doctors how they arrived at their "maximum" numbers, most would say that they have no idea. More often than not, their appointment books have actually predetermined the maximum capacity of their practices – effectively putting a lid on growth.

Every practice eventually reaches a point of equilibrium at which growth ceases and volume levels off. This point is different for each practice, but quite often, it is reached when the slots in the appointment book are filled, and this usually has nothing to do with the doctor's or the staff's ability to see more patients. When serving as a resident, I observed one practice that booked patients every half hour. The doctor had a stellar reputation and was booked weeks in advance. One day, he decided to change his booking from every half hour to every twenty minutes. Instead of seeing sixteen patients a day, he now saw twenty-four (with no difficulty). The volume and income of this practice increased 50% virtually "overnight." Interestingly, this practitioner never went any further; he never considered the possibility of booking patients every fifteen minutes. Rather, he now saw his schedule as "full" at twenty-four. Even if you do not seek to fill all empty time slots, the more spaces you have available to you, the more flexible you can be. I have seen some practices that have unknowingly reduced volume over time simply by filling time slots with notes, thus reducing space for potential patients. When you have "extra" slots in your book, you can use several, as a block, to schedule longer appointments for specific services. Regardless of the type of appointment book you currently use, if you want your practice to grow, your "book" must have more slots available than numbers of patients you could possibly see on your busiest day.

Overbooking Works

Many practices are overly focused on no-shows, often resulting in scheduling policies that waste staff time, alienate patients, and can lead to lower productivity due to "under-booking." While it is important to generate no-show and cancellation reports so that these patients can be tracked and followed-up on, practices that call all patients in advance to remind them of their appointments or threaten to charge fees for missed appointments are typically doing this to "help" with productivity. They are attempting to assure that the doctor will not be idle. While it makes sense to call the small number of patients who are scheduled for surgery or lengthy visits (this does tend to assure they will be on time and help the doctor to stay on schedule), it is generally unproductive to call all patients. A percentage will still cancel or not show up, and patients scheduled for shorter visits are typically seen as they arrive at the office anyway, reducing the possibility that any late patient will put the doctor behind.

While there are software programs that can automatically call patients to remind them of appointments, a better "solution" is to overbook patients, based on the practice's historic no-show and cancellation rates. Two University of Colorado researchers published a study (which won the 2007 Best Paper Award from *Decision Sciences*) showing that overbooking increases productivity. If a practice is efficiently managed, this practice also creates opportunities for growth. The worst-case scenario occurs on a day when every patient shows up; making patient waits longer than average on that specific day. While there are worse problems a practice can have, when this occurs consistently, it signals that the practice should hire additional staff or consider the possibility of taking on an associate or physician extender. Ultimately, a doctor needs to recognize that medical practices are similar to airlines in that, even when there are "empty seats," the total cost of the "flight" remains the same. Empty seats result in lower profitability, and for this reason, focus should be on strategies that will insure that seats are filled.

How to Continue Revenue Growth when You Are Booked Solid

The fundamental economic goal sought by all industries is to maximize profit, not volume. This requires seeking an optimum, rather than a maximum, volume. The goal should not be to maximize volume because operational efficiency declines as volume nears maximum capacity. Random hourly and daily volume fluctuations cannot be accommodated when a practice is at maximum capacity, and as volume nears maximum, inefficiencies develop at an accelerated rate, resulting in disproportionately high costs, lost revenues, and low quality. As a company or practice nears maximum volume, its decision makers must decide whether it will be more profitable to add capacity or "selectively" reduce volume – an answer that will be different for each business within the same industry.

A useful axiom to keep in mind when making this type of decision is one used in the consulting industry. Simply stated: as volume reaches capacity, one must be prepared to give up the bottom 15% of business in order to increase revenue. Eliminating the bottom 15% creates *capacity* for new business, and this can be in focused areas – areas in which the provider is especially skilled and/or has greatest interest. Because the bottom 15% of revenue is frequently generated by a volume that is disproportionately higher than 15%, a greater capacity than might be expected will be "freed up" for revenue growth, not to mention that opportunities for reducing the costs associated with excess capacity will also be created.

If we were to apply this axiom to a medical practice, we might state it as: the bottom 15% of a practice's revenue may, or may not, be generated by the lowest paying third party payer currently under consideration for discontinuation by the practice. Perhaps that bottom 15% is the result of specific diagnoses or types of service.

A practice that is below capacity and has doctor(s) and staff with significant idle time may not have a bottom 15% to give up. In these cases, reducing volume (even low-paying volume) is likely to reduce profit. On the other hand, a practice that is near capacity has the option of increasing efficiency or turning any lower paying business over to an associate who is not practicing near capacity, rather than eliminating the business from the practice. It is important to consider the impact that such a decision will have on referral sources and profit. Remember, there is no "one size fits all" solution.

In addition to reimbursement rates, an equally significant factor to consider when making a decision to keep, or give up, a segment of patients is whether or not the source of the bottom 15% of revenue provides a satisfying type of work. Low fees are one aspect to consider, but many doctors volunteer time in "free clinics" and foreign lands simply because they enjoy treating certain conditions. If the type of work is satisfying, or enjoyable, even a low paying contract is more profitable than volunteering time for free. The point is that if a doctor dislikes providing a specific type of service, or finds working under a specific contract aggravating, low fees are only one reason for giving up that contract. These patients can either be referred out or seen by another doctor within the same practice who is more adept at, or enjoys treating, their specific conditions. In most cases, increased patient satisfaction and higher profit result from taking this kind of action, and one reason for this is that, once this 15% of work is "given up", the doctor now has more time to focus on the things that s/he prefers treating and is best at.

The number one reason most often cited by doctors for holding on to the bottom 15% of revenue is their fear of losing income. Support for the argument of eliminating this bottom 15% can be found in the "old-days" of pre-managed care – the 60s and 70s. At that time, many doctors worked six days a week. Those who wanted to spend more time with their families feared that if they discontinued Saturday hours (or hired a doctor to see patients on Saturdays), they would lose income; however, Bob Levoy and other noted practice management "gurus" who lectured at the time could cite no cases of doctors who had lost income following discontinuation of Saturday hours. Interestingly, this drop from working six days, to five, is statistically similar to dropping the bottom 15% of business. I have yet to see a busy practice that has eliminated the bottom 15% of its patients end up being less profitable.

If you are "booked solid" and contemplating opting out of a specific contract, it is a worthwhile exercise to examine all your sources of revenue and identify the "bottom 15%" before making that final decision. Once you know what this bottom 15% includes, you will be making a more informed decision – one that can lead to optimized volume and greater patient satisfaction while, at the same time, building a more profitable practice with a more enjoyable work environment. If the only problem you have with a contract is that it is low paying, simply knowing that you can walk away from it without losing income will put you in a much stronger position for negotiating a new, fairer rate for that contract.

After decreasing patient volume, you will have more time to treat patients and can seek an increase in your volume of services. Typically, a doctor seeing a high number of patients is rushed and, therefore, has time to focus only on "fixing" each patient's chief concern – often overlooking, or putting off until "later," the examination and treatment of secondary complaints. This results in the delivery of fewer services per patient and, hence, lost revenue. This also leads to a drop in patient satisfaction because it is quite common that a patient's secondary complaint is actually a chronic problem that s/he has been putting off for some time – something that necessitated the development of a more acute problem to even motivate him/her enough to schedule an appointment. Any new "found time" created by a drop in patient volume offers the doctor an opportunity to discuss and schedule appropriate treatment for all concerns – resulting in a truly satisfied patient.

If you want a useful benchmark for comparing yourself with your peers – in this area of treating secondary complaints – know that you are probably not following up on these complaints and have an opportunity for improvement if your ratio of CPT codes billed, per patient visit, is closer to 1.0 than to 2.0. Large groups have an additional opportunity open to them for increasing their number of services, and this is the opportunity to offer ancillary services. This works particularly well for large groups because these services typically require a large patient volume to support the additional overhead they generate. It is important to note that increasing service volume will result in satisfied patients and increased profit only if the practice is simultaneously focusing on efficiency, adequate capacity (optimum staffing ratios and number of treatment rooms) and effective time management (including a significant focus on appropriate scheduling of patient appointments).

Consider Offering Same-Day Appointments

Patients value immediate access; don't you when you are the patient? Because today's family schedules are complicated, we value flexibility, and for those seeking growth, this is certainly something to consider. If you are concerned that open access might suddenly overload your schedule, you might consider conducting a controlled test. Keep a limited number of appointment slots set aside for patients who call-in, requesting same-day appointments. Note: this requires that you have a sufficient number of slots in your "book." If your trial shows promise, you can take this as signal that you should adopt this as a permanent policy. Begin preparing for growth!

The policy of offering same-day appointments presents several advantages. You would be surprised how much staff time can be saved by not having to explain to prospective patients how busy your practice is and why there are no appointments available on the days or at the times that work best for them. Obviously, this type of dialogue will not help to grow any practice, and it might even be a prescription for decline. Being booked weeks in advance is not the "sign of excellence" that some doctors feel it to be – rather it tends to indicate to patients that either 1) the practice is not managed effectively or 2) the doctor does not care about them. With open time slots, scheduling conversations change to, "What time would you like to come in?" Again, this not only helps create growth, but it eliminates much of the stress associated with scheduling, allowing staff to feel good about meeting patient needs (which is probably why they went into medicine in the first place). This type of scheduling also creates opportunities for strategies such as e-scheduling. Open slots which are designated for same day appointments can be made available to patients who would appreciate the convenience of scheduling their own appointments online. This not only offers a marketing advantage, but it requires no staff time, and when coupled with decentralized scheduling, further reduces the classic, front desk bottleneck.

Your Paper Appointment Book Is Outdated

An appointment book is used to manage time – the most important resource a doctor has. Since his/her time is limited, planning its use is critically important to all areas of a practice – improvement in quality and productivity, cost reduction, successful treatment outcomes, and patient satisfaction. Of these areas, patient satisfaction is the most important to overall practice success. The Pay for Quality and value-based reimbursement programs currently being initiated by third party payers will be looking especially hard at patient satisfaction, which they see as one of the factors patients and employers value most. As a practitioner, you should know that every patient satisfaction survey conducted in the past thirty years has confirmed the following as the top four patient concerns: 1) access to an office, 2) the amount of time spent waiting during an office visit, 3) the thoroughness with which the doctor listens and explains, and 4) the efficiency and courtesy of office staff. All of these issues are "time" related – dependent on an efficient workflow plan, and this requires the effective use of a well-designed appointment "book."

Using an appointment book as a practice improvement tool is a concept that has interested me for a long time. In fact, I delivered my first lecture on appointment scheduling in 1975. At the time, the standard appointment book was the "week-at-a-glance" model, which contained one vertical column for each day of the week, with the columns broken into fifteen-minute intervals. Most doctors starting out in practice received this appointment book for free from one of the supply companies, and they sent a new one each year. Many doctors simply continued using these books throughout their careers, in spite of the fact that, as their practices became busier and more complex, the use of a single, vertical column for booking an entire day afforded almost no flexibility. There was no space allotted for planning ahead or managing workflow, which often proved a hindrance to patients attempting to access the practice, produced long waits during office visits, and ultimately, limited practice growth.

Through the utilization of ever-advancing technology, appointment scheduling has come a long way since 1975; however, few of the doctors using this new technology have captured all of its potential advantages. In fact, many practices currently using "advanced" technology actually scheduled appointments just as effectively when they were using their old paper appointment books. Since effectively applied appointment scheduling serves well as both an operational and a strategic tool, it is important to take a close look at the current technology and determine how to use it most advantageously. Knowing which of its features are important to incorporate into your practice and applying those features appropriately can make a significant positive impact on multiple areas of your practice.

Buying Scheduling Software: Which One to Choose?

Don't get lost in the "bells and whistles" of competing software brands. Most doctors find the "latest and greatest" features of technology distracting, believing that these are what will make the difference in the efficiency and productivity of their practices. For example, doctors often ask questions such as, "Does the software work by touch screen, key board, mouse clicks, or voice activation?" In reality, the data entry method that is "best" for any one practice depends mostly on personal preference. These software features should have little to do with a practice's ultimate decision as to which system to buy because good hardware and software programs offer all of these choices, and none of them has much to do with how the software will be used to improve practice workflow.

In order to improve office productivity and efficiency, what you ultimately want is for all practice computers to be networked so that when information is entered into any one computer in the office (whether by touch screen, keyboard, mouse clicks, or voice activation), it is instantly available on all of the others. It should be possible to perform any office transaction from any computer terminal in the network, including those in satellite offices, at home, or in the hospital. When selecting technology, remember that it is these networking and accessibility capabilities that ultimately determine the system's merit and not the "bells and whistles" – features which are mostly issues of personal preference.

Your scheduling program should "look like" an appointment book. Easy visualization is a feature of paper appointment books that makes them "simple" to use. A scheduler using an electronic book can find open appointments for a specific day, week, or month "at a glance," and the patient's name can be entered in seconds. Also, when multiple doctors practice together, their individual appointment schedules can be viewed side-by-side. This makes "same-day" appointment slots easier to find; it is easy to see which doctor is most available at the time needed.

This may seem a relatively obvious scheduling format to employ; yet, some electronic programs use formats that are radically different. Some display a demographic screen to the person entering an appointment; she/he does not actually view the schedule. Also, with some software, once the appointment date and time have been determined, the process of actually entering the patient's appointment requires a lengthy and time consuming process of mouse clicks, tabs, and keystrokes. The features of paper appointment books that worked well, i.e. the ability to quickly find and schedule an appointment, are often omitted in these electronic schedulers. Rather than improving or enhancing the process, these "new and improved" electronic processes can be unnecessarily more complex, less intuitive, and less effective.

An electronic schedule should offer the flexibility of multiple views, depending on what specific task you wish to accomplish. Sometimes it is important to view one doctor's schedule for a specific day, at others, for an entire week or month, and yet, at other times, you might want to view multiple doctors, or multiple locations, side-by-side. All of these options should be instantly possible, and all should be presented in formats that are easily visualized and quick to access and use.

There are seemingly endless ways to customize an electronic schedule. One designed for a multi-doctor practice should be customizable for each doctor in terms of appointment length and the number of columns s/he needs for double or triple booking. Every scheduling program must make it easy to select an appointment time and enter a patient's name directly onto the schedule with only a few "clicks." Visual enhancements are another plus; they can prevent errors and promote efficiency because they increase the amount of "at a glance" information available to the scheduler. These enhancements include such things as multiple color slots for signaling various information – such as: the type of appointment, an indication that the patient has been called confirming his/her appointment, or confirmation that insurance has been verified. All of these enhancements make a scheduling program more effective and easier to use.

Finally, in order to achieve maximum benefit and efficiency from computerized scheduling, the appointment software must be fully integrated with practice management and clinical software. This assures that all information is shared and linked, thus avoiding double entry into separate databases. When a patient checks-in, an audit trail is begun so that it can be determined at the end of the day whether documentation in the patient's chart was completed, the patient checked-out, and his/her charges were entered. Simply "clicking" on the schedule at the patient's name should bring up any information that is needed, such as his/her electronic medical record or financial, demographic, or insurance information.

Seven Ways to Improve Your Scheduling Process Using Technology

1. Network your schedule

The ability to use an electronic schedule enterprise wide offers a significant advantage over a paper schedule. When a system is enterprise wide, appointments can be made from the front desk, a central call center, a treatment room, a doctor or nurse's desk, or from any one office to another in a separate geographic location. This type of flexibility is critical to effective management, and looking ahead to a future where mergers and the formation of larger groups is likely to become the norm, an effective and efficient system-wide scheduling process will be crucial to success. This type of technology creates the opportunity to schedule appointments both where and when the process best fits into the workflow. This also allows scheduling to be performed by *any* staff member, based on his/her availability. A process designed in this way immediately accommodates random variations in call volume or scheduling, facilitating a smooth workflow.

Perhaps the most significant improvement that enterprise wide scheduling has to offer is the ability to schedule return-patient appointments from treatment rooms. This one feature alone reduces the checkout, re-scheduling bottleneck that regularly occurs at the front desk. The future schedule flows more smoothly because the clinical personnel making return appointments are steeped in the knowledge necessary for the most accurate scheduling (i.e. the appropriate call-back time and length of appointment that will be needed). When clinical personnel become involved in scheduling follow-up visits, workflow is changed in a way that expands office capacity. For example, a "five minute check" gets scheduled in front of a twenty five minute patient consult visit, assuring that the patient and the treatment room scheduled for the "quick check" are not tied up for an unnecessary, extra, twenty minutes – a true win-win situation for both the doctor and the patients.

2. Use time stamps to improve workflow

Much of the value to be gained from an electronic schedule is derived from the opportunity it provides for communicating information between various locations in an office. When patients are checked in, their "charts" should be time-stamped in "real time." This information is made immediately available in the clinical areas. When the doctor views his/her personal schedule from any clinical area, it should be obvious which patients have arrived at the office (usually by the patients' names changing color) and at what times they arrived. This gives the doctors and clinical staff the information necessary for best managing workflow, hour by hour, as the day unfolds.

Think of how many times your practice experiences a pause in work, when clinical personnel and doctors in the back office are standing around waiting for patients to "arrive" while several may have already done so but are still being "processed" at the front desk. When patient arrival is displayed in the clinical area, in real time, a clinical staff member can go to the front and escort the patient to a treatment room so that the doctor can begin treatment immediately and not "suddenly" have three patients at once. When things are bogging down at the front desk, this "stamped" check-in time alerts the doctor and back office staff, providing them with the opportunity to decide who should be seen next.

Time-stamping should be done at various stages as the patient progresses through the office: 1) when the patient arrives, 2) when s/he is admitted to a treatment room, and 3) at checkout. Using this information, the practice can produce objective reports that measure patient waits, and these reports, in turn, can be used to evaluate whether efforts to reduce wait times are succeeding.

3. Automate each doctor's scheduling preferences

The larger your group, the more difficult it is to schedule properly without the use of electronic scheduling. Each doctor in a practice has unique preferences for scheduling patients, and it is difficult for personnel to remember each physician's preferences every time a patient is being scheduled. "Preferences" might include such things as: 1) limiting the number of new patients to one, each hour, 2) designating a specific day for surgery, 3) limiting HMO patients from a specific plan to a specified number, per day, 4) allowing only certain types of visits to be booked at the end of the day – or just prior to the lunch hour, or 5) designating certain conditions that the doctor does not treat. A rules-based appointment schedule that allows such preferences to be programmed into the system decreases the potential for inaccurate bookings. Without rules-based scheduling, mistakes are often discovered after it is too late – when the patient arrives for his/her "flawed" appointment.

I do have a word of caution regarding scheduling rules, and this is that having too many can be just as bad as having no rules at all – especially as the number of doctors in a group increases. I once consulted for a G.I. practice that had four doctors and four schedulers. This seemed excessive to me as the practice had one-third the volume of others I had observed that were able to function quite well using only one scheduler. Upon examination, we discovered that each doctor had slightly different scheduling "rules" – making it difficult for one person to schedule appointments for all of them without making mistakes. After identifying and evaluating several dozen of these rules, each used by at least one of the four doctors, the group determined that only two of these were actually important enough to preserve. Following simplification of this list, the number of schedulers was reduced to two, and these two were able to do a better job than the four had done previously.

Once rules are entered into the system, a scheduler cannot make an appointment that breaks those rules. If need be, a rule can be over-ridden, but only by someone with the security clearance necessary for "breaking a rule." For example, if a doctor wants to see a maximum of one new patient, per hour, a scheduler attempting to add a new patient thirty minutes following another new patient might only be allowed to accomplish this by first receiving clearance from the doctor. When "rules-based" software is not used, mistakes are common, and reducing their frequency requires that you hire additional personnel.

4. Maximize doctor effort

There is a significant discrepancy between the amount of time a patient spends in the treatment room and the time that the doctor spends in the room with that patient. For example, assume that a doctor has three patients booked between 2:00pm and 3:00pm. One is new to the practice and will be in the treatment room for forty minutes, and the other two are follow-up visits, each of whom will be in a treatment room for twenty minutes. These three patients will "tie up" treatment rooms for a total of eighty minutes. Assume that the time the doctor spends with the new patient will be twenty minutes and that each follow up visit will require five minutes of his/her time. This is only a total of thirty minutes. In this example, even though patients "fill" the entire hour from 2:00 to 3:00, only fifty percent of the physician's time is actually being utilized in that hour. Viewed from an "efficiency perspective," fifty percent of the physician's potential "effort" is being wasted.

An ideal appointment book will monitor the percentage of each physician's effort being scheduled, maximizing productivity. Once an individual doctor's "effort" is 100% scheduled, a visual sign (such as a color change) will occur to signal that this doctor's maximum effort has been reached. The scheduler can see at a glance which time slots have not yet reached 100%, and patients can be scheduled at those remaining times – ones that will work best for both the doctor and the patients.

5. Maximize your resources

Some patient visits require specific resources that are in limited supply, and these should be scheduled accordingly. For example, a patient may need an ultrasound exam for which the office has only one machine. When this patient is scheduled, the ultrasound equipment resource should be linked to his/her appointment so that another patient requiring this same resource will not be scheduled at the same time. Other specific resources might include 1) a specific room, such as one for X-Rays, casting, or minor surgical procedures, 2) specific equipment, such as ultrasound, fluoroscope, or laser, or 3) specific personnel, such as a physical therapist, a cast tech, or a medical assistant who has a unique skill. Assurance that no resources will be double-booked reduces delays in patient visits and improves overall office workflow.

6. Use appointment notes to reduce errors

Appointment notes can serve as an important tool for preventing errors and making a patient's visit proceed smoothly. While most electronic scheduling systems have areas for notes regarding a patient's diagnosis, it is important that they also provide "pop-up notes" to alert the doctor and staff when there is something important to know about a specific patient *before* making an appointment, *during* the appointment, or *after* the appointment, when rescheduling. These pop-up notes can alert the doctor and staff to such matters as 1) potential drug "conflicts," 2) the need to inform a patient not to eat or drink after midnight prior to an office visit, 3) the necessity for a referral or authorization for the patient's further treatment, 4) any special patient needs, i.e. "requires a wheelchair" or "is hard of hearing," or 5) the fact that the patient's account is seriously past due and that s/he should speak with the billing office before scheduling his/her next appointment. All such reminders cause the work to flow more smoothly and help reduce errors, thus increasing office efficiency and productivity.

7. Multi tasking features help your receptionist

Because many medical practices require that their receptionist at the front desk be capable of multi-tasking (answer the phone, make appointments, input demographic data, and check patients in and out), it is important for the appointment book to have features that facilitate these tasks. An appointment book that can be used to scan insurance cards, driver's licenses, and other patient-related documentation and then integrate that information into the system, eliminates the need for filing paper records in a chart, making it no longer necessary for schedulers to pull charts and review this documentation when appointing a patient. Other helpful features include: the ability to alert the receptionist to co-payment amounts, automatically attach co-payments to the dates-of-service, and designate a form of payment that will stay with each date-of-service, regardless of any subsequent change in coverage. If the receptionist is making appointments over the phone or making return appointments for patients exiting the office, the ability to search for "first available" by date, time of day, provider, and/or location facilitates this scheduling process. Obviously, the greater the number of doctors practicing together, the more helpful these features become.

Chapter 7

Get the Most Out of Your EMR

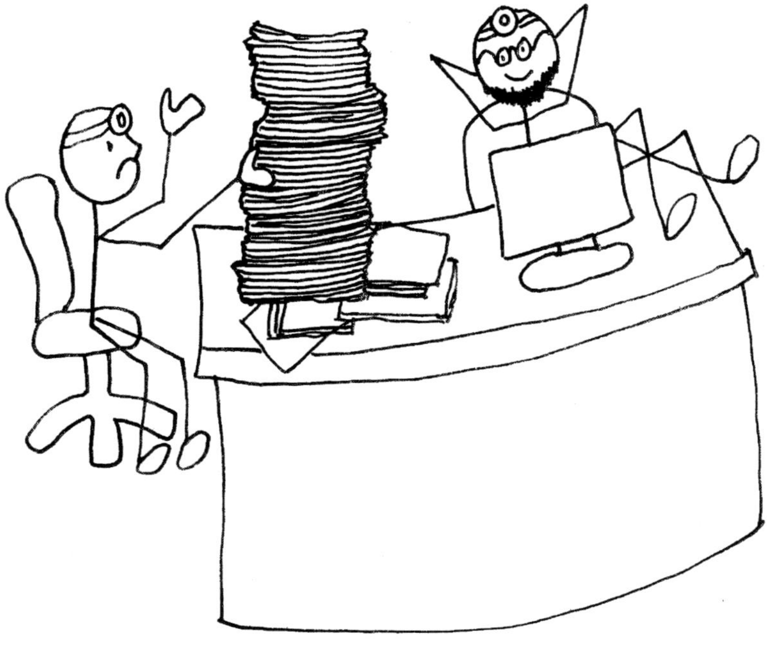

The Benefits of Going Paperless

In today's price competitive environment, companies strive to find ways to do things better, for less. When healthcare leaders first began to look for ways of accomplishing this, the elimination of paper seemed an obvious place to start. Efforts to eliminate paper began decades ago, and in spite of the multitude of technological improvements since that time, physician adoption of paperless technology has been slow. While a "paperless" process does not automatically lead to efficiencies that increase quality and lower costs, the implementation of an electronic medical record (one part of the "paperless process") is something that does – as long as all necessary efficiency principles are incorporated into the process and the users address, in advance, all the goals expected to be achieved from the software.

In October of 2000, *Modern Healthcare* presented a poll showing that 39% of physicians who were resolved to eliminate paper medical records intended to implement an EMR within the year. Tellingly, however, several years later, fewer than 5% were actually employing an EMR. It is likely that more physicians would use EMRs if they realized the magnitude of the negative impact that paper medical records can have on the costs of their medical practices and the quality of the treatment they render.

Consider the following statistics compiled over a twenty-year period by groups that include the AMA, the U.S. General Accounting Office, and the Medical Record Institute:

- Percent of patient encounters at which a doctor is unable to access the patient's medical records: 30%
- Percent of physician's time spent writing, dictating, or searching for information in medical records: 38%
- Percent of times a patient's diagnosis is not recorded in the medical record: 40%
- Percent of times a patient's chief complaint is not recorded in the medical record: 27%
- Percent of staff members in a hospital who may need to access the same patient's medical record at any given time: 22%

- Percent of staff time spent retrieving, moving, searching through, and re-filing medical records to answer patient questions: 16.5%
- Percent of physician "order entry" errors that a computerized system has been shown to prevent: 50%
- Average weight of a paper medical record: 1.5 pounds

Electronic medical records offer a "simple" solution to each of these problems, and when implemented properly, they simultaneously decrease costs and increase quality. By no means does all of this happen automatically. Without the proper application of efficiency principles, a paperless medical records process can be utilized just as inefficiently as a paper based one. Most doctors initially used "stand alone" (non-integrated) EMR systems. These functioned primarily as what I would refer to as dictation replacements. Even though these systems reduced dictation costs, doctors continued to print out their medical records and employ them in much the same way as before – capturing none of the cost and quality benefits achievable through an integrated EMR.

The above list of statistics reveals the significant opportunities to be captured through use of an EMR. Additional opportunities include: streamlined operations, timely access to medical information, fewer medical errors, the opportunity to offer enhanced patient education, improved risk management, clinical outcomes reporting, intelligent prompting, and lower costs. The most immediate benefits are the cost savings and quality improvement opportunities attained simply through the reduction of the mechanical inefficiencies inherent in the workflow of a paper based process. In particular, an effective EMR creates the potential for substantial cost savings through reduction of staff numbers – and, thereby, a lowering of total staff salaries. Studies have shown that 16.5% of staff time in a medical practice is spent dealing with issues brought about because a practice is using paper records. This translates to one full-time salary – one staff person out of every six – essentially being spent on "wasted time" – time for which the practice receives no productive or financial benefit. The EMR eliminates these wasted steps and, along with them, the need for this additional salary expense.

In the near future, integration of an EMR into a medical practice will be essential to addressing the important healthcare quality and reimbursement issues now at the forefront of healthcare debates. They will, for instance, make it easier for doctors to receive reimbursement under measures such as pay for performance and pay for quality. Utilizing an electronic health record can help practitioners provide higher quality care, improve their operations, save costs today, and prepare doctors for electronic compliance in the future.

EMR Is More than Just "Electronic Paper"

In a 1991 paper, Stanford University economic historian, Paul David, compared the diffusion of computer technology to the replacement of steam engines by smaller electric motors. With the initial introduction of the smaller, more efficient, electric motors, industrial productivity actually decreased. David concluded that this was because factory managers first used them as substitute steam engines, much as the first computers were used as substitute typewriters and adding machines. Electric motors first made a positive impact on productivity when factory managers realized that the principal advantage of these smaller and lighter engines was that they could be taken to where the work was. After creatively re-thinking the way these new machines could be used, productivity gains followed. In other words, implementation of this new technology only created gains in the workplace when the workflow was simultaneously redesigned.

A parallel exists between the way these electric motors were eventually used and the way that we can effectively use computer technology to achieve quality and productivity gains in our practices. With computers, as with electric motors, the primary problem has not been the tool, but rather, how the "tool" has been inserted into our workflow. Since information can be delivered anywhere in an office through the use of computer technology, we need to take advantage of the fact that tasks can now be performed at the places in the workflow where they best "fit" – where they make the most sense. Unfortunately, in spite of major advances in technology, computers are still not being used this way in most medical practices. The majority of tasks continue to be performed in traditional locations, whether or not those locations make the most sense.

Especially useful tools in the technology arsenal, EMRs have been ready for prime time since 1994 and have been added to many software programs; however, their effective use requires not only a change in office workflow, but also a change in the way that software companies sell, train, implement, and support their software. In most cases, this has not occurred in practices or at software companies, resulting in implementations that have achieved suboptimal outcomes.

In 1999, I accompanied several physicians to the annual TEPR (Towards Electronic Patient Records) meeting. These doctors, who were in the process of evaluating electronic medical records software for their group, wanted to learn more about EMRs so that they would be capable of making an educated purchase decision. Each physician attended thirty lectures and spent every free moment in the exhibit hall viewing software demos and interacting with exhibitors who presented over 200 EMR programs. They also spoke with customers who were using the various programs. By the end of an intensive week, this group was even more confused and further from making a decision than they had been before. How is a physician to evaluate these many systems?

I was a speaker at this TEPR meeting, and I attended many of the lectures. I recall many speakers discussing "failures" which had resulted from events that, in my opinion, could easily have been predicted and avoided ahead of time. Even several well-known large medical groups experienced these failures, groups that had the advantages of adequate capital for investment, full-time managers, information technology personnel, and outside consultants. Knowing this, I wondered, "How can physicians who practice in smaller groups make 'correct' purchasing decisions, experience successful implementations, or achieve the quality and profitability goals they expect from their investments in technology?" Attempting to answer this question and help you avoid a failed implementation requires a discussion of areas that may seem unrelated. They all are, however, potential barriers to achieving successful implementation and positive long-term outcomes. Let us take a look at some relevant issues that will help you make a more informed decision and avoid pitfalls that might prevent your achieving effective implementation.

Take the Engine to Where the Work Is

It is well recognized that locating computer terminals in patient treatment rooms is necessary for effectively integrating the EMR into patient care. What often goes unrecognized is that the implementation of an electronic medical record simultaneously creates the opportunity to convert inefficient, dependent series processes into highly efficient, parallel ones. Each new terminal creates an *external* "parallel lane," enabling doctors and support staff who are temporarily idled throughout a busy day to utilize their idle time effectively, even enabling them to assist staff at distant locations where bottlenecks are occurring and temporary help is needed.

Fully integrating an electronic medical record, appointment scheduler, billing software, e-prescription process, and all other practice management features is comparable to adding *internal* parallel lanes which, in addition to the external "parallel lanes" created by additional computer terminals, further enhance the opportunity to convert series processes into parallel ones. These internal lanes enable multiple software related transactions to occur simultaneously – in parallel with one another. For example, when a prescription is written, it is legible, dosing errors are avoided, and the software simultaneously searches for allergies and potential harmful interactions with other medications the patient may already be taking, alerting the doctor to any problems. The prescription can then be submitted to the pharmacy, on-line, with instructions printed out for the patient – reinforcing what the doctor has already discussed with him/her.

These previously unrecognized "parallel opportunities" to be obtained from EMR implementation can be captured at no additional expense and in the same amount of time as is required simply for effective integration of an EMR into a practice. Locating these additional computer terminals throughout a medical office further enables doctors and staff to perform work where it makes the most sense in the workflow – often vastly different locations from where this work has been performed in the past. These external and internal parallel lanes created at the time of EMR implementation projects, in combination with the ability to perform work where it makes the most sense, are what will enable a medical practice to effectively redesign workflow in ways that create the kinds of efficiencies that lead to higher quality and lower costs.

Set Concrete Goals for EMR Implementation

We intuitively know that any project should begin with a goal in mind. The problem is that most physicians set goals for their EMR projects that are either inappropriate or too narrow, dooming them from the start. The stated goal may be simply, "I want my practice to be paperless," or "I want to be on an EMR." As mentioned above, many physicians see an EMR as a dictation replacement, rather than a tool for decision support, error reduction, efficiency improvement, and storage of searchable data – which, in the near future, will be useable for evidence based medicine. This searchable data will be used for improving patient outcomes and delivering the type of coordinated care that employers, payers, and the government expect, care which will improve treatment quality and slow the rising costs of healthcare. A goal such as "paperlessness" or "dictation replacement" can be achieved by any EMR project; however, a practice can become paperless or be using an EMR and still be as inefficient as before – certainly not prepared for the future of evidence based medicine with its quality initiatives such as "pay for performance." Setting narrow goals results in missing out on the more sweeping productive outcomes that can be achieved through use of an EMR – outcomes such as improvement in treatment quality, increased productivity and profitability, greater efficiency, higher patient satisfaction, reduction of errors, and creation of more time for doctors to spend with patients.

Embarking upon a technology "improvement project" without a clear, substantial goal in mind helps explain the "typical experience" that Bill Gates relates in his 1991 book *Business @ the Speed of Thought*. In this book he states, "The typical company is getting only 20% of the benefits possible from technology." This is certainly the case in most medical practices. I believe the primary reason for this is that doctors set goals for their technology that are too narrow – ones that do not adequately address the issue of workflow efficiency. Since the amount of time and money you will need to invest in order to achieve multiple goals from your EMR project is the same as you would need to achieve just one, you should make certain that you define all of your goals from the start – challenging yourself and your chosen software company to figure out just how these goals will be achieved *before* your purchase decision is made and your implementation plan put into action.

You may want to seek help in setting and achieving your goals. The most difficult requirement of successful technology and EMR implementation is that the person who is going to evaluate the purchase of technology, plan the project, and execute it successfully must have a diverse set of skills – including knowledge of clinical medicine, technology, industrial engineering, medical economics, project management, billing and coding, and policies and procedures. Developing and applying these skills effectively is also maximized by experience. Most physicians who write about EMRs have the necessary clinical knowledge, but they are typically writing about something they have read, or they are basing their recommendations on the limited experience they have gained from implementing and using a specific product in their own practices.

Most physicians use technology "experts" or software company sales people as advisors. Those in sales, however, not only have a conflict of interest, but there is a well known "disconnect" between the software sales people who make the promises and the project management teams whose job it is to eventually implement that software and deliver on those promises. Also, while technology "experts" are essential to this process, they are not the ones who should be giving advice on product selection, redesigning workflow, or determining how implementation should be directed at the achievement of specific goals. This would be comparable to asking the manufacturer of power surgical equipment which surgical procedure to perform and how to perform it. My advice is that you meet with a *project management team* composed of office staff members along with implementation representatives from the software company before making your software decision. Make sure that they all understand your goals and the actual capabilities of the software program and can assist in designing an implementation plan which will deliver on "promised" results.

How to Choose EMR Software

The most common reason given by doctors for putting off purchase of an EMR is that they are waiting to be told what the "best" software is. When I am asked what this "magic" software might be, I reply with, "What is the best word processing software – Microsoft Word or WordPerfect? They can both do the job. The more relevant question is, do you know how to write?" "Writing well" will take a combination of the word processing software, writing skill, and effective support for helping the user to become a better writer – some of which must come in the form of value-added services from the software company. Likewise, there are many EMR programs that can "do the job," but the companies behind them must provide assistance and on-going support that will enable the user to achieve higher quality and profitability in his/her practice.

Much of the software selection process comes down to one important question, "What are you trying to accomplish with the program?" If your goal is simply to replace dictation or become "paperless," almost any program will do. If you are also looking to improve workflow, reduce costs, improve quality, increase productivity and profitability, you must understand that, as when comparing Word Perfect to Microsoft Word, medical software programs are merely enablers; they will not, on their own, automatically improve a practice anymore than a word processing program will make a person a better writer. It is how you apply the chosen software that will make the difference.

Help is available to assist doctors in narrowing the field when they are attempting to find "better" EMR software programs. Given the future needs for physician collaboration and assurance that the electronic health records in their practices and the hospitals they use will be able to communicate with one another in a seamless fashion (interoperability), it would make sense to check the list of products certified by the Authorized Testing and Certification Bodies (ATCBs) – selected by the Office of the National Coordinator for Health information Technology (ONC). Currently, there are five ATCBs on the list, including Surescripts, LLC, SLI Global Solutions, InfoGard Laboratories, Inc., Certification Commission for Health Information Technology, and the Drummond Group, Inc. Because the certification process is quickly evolving – as are the number of certificated products, selection criteria, and the certifying bodies themselves – it would be prudent to seek the most up-to-date information about certification immediately prior to initiating your search to find an electronic health record that meets your needs as well as the coordinated care and quality needs of future healthcare delivery.

Think when Purchasing Your EMR

The fact that there is a certification process in place is still not, on its own, going to ensure that a doctor achieves a successful implementation in his/her practice or that there will be any efficiency or quality gains as a result of "successful" implementation of EMR software. Two certified products were featured as "implementation failures" in an April 7, 2006, *Medical Economics* article entitled, "Why EHRs Falter." Again, most "failures" do not come about because the technology is "bad," but rather, because practices often automate existing processes without simultaneously redesigning workflow to address the bottlenecks, variation, and waste issues discussed in chapters two and three.

Earlier, I worked with a medical group that was considering one of the certified products cited as a "failure" in the *Medical Economics* article. When one of the doctors, who understood workflow and efficiency concepts, asked the salesperson whether the software could be used from treatment rooms to schedule return visits, she replied, "Why would you want to do that?" She went on to ask, "How do you do this now?" with the physician replying, "The way we do it now isn't working." The doctor was suggesting that the practice use the software to enable one of many workflow processes proven to significantly improve a practice's patient satisfaction ratings, capacity, and profitability levels. The problem is that the salesperson did not understand how locating the technology and EMR in treatment rooms would revolutionize this practice's workflow; instead, she simply wanted to make this sale and move on to the next. Keep in mind that a sales person is rewarded for making sales, not for achieving improved practice performance. As a result, many "failures" occur; this is not because the software is inadequate but because proper implementation goals have not been set ahead of time.

The software sales and implementation process is also flawed in that it has not adapted to the introduction of EMRs into the "package." Traditionally, pre-sales discussions took place between business office staff and salespeople because business staff members were the ones who primarily would be using the software for day-to-day operations. Physicians and clinical nursing staff were basically "out of the picture" because the technology was not going to be widely introduced into the clinical areas. This technology was not going to change their existing workflow. As we have discussed, however, for an EMR to be successfully implemented, the workflow of *all* staff members will need to be changed. Unfortunately, the sales process has not significantly changed to reflect this reality.

It is impossible to implement EMR software effectively without involving the doctors. I find that success is virtually assured if all physicians are fully committed and directly involved with the selection, implementation plan, and its execution. If they are not, the EMR never becomes fully functional because only some of the doctors and clinical staff end up utilizing it to its full capability. This is the rule rather than the exception.

Even at the point in time at which software company surveys claimed that at least 30% of practices were on EMRs, in my experience, I found that fewer than 5% actually were, and even fewer were using EMRs in a meaningful way or at any level close to their maximum capabilities. Approximately 30% of practices at the time had purchased software programs that included EMRs, and if these EMRs were being used at all, only one physician in the group typically was doing so. Unless all doctors in a group are using the EMR, the costs associated with dictation, maintaining paper charts, and manually entering superbill data will continue because the practice must maintain parallel paper processes for the medical records and superbills of the doctors who are not "on" the software. Since early 2011, when doctors were first offered stimulus money as an incentive for utilizing a certified EMR program in a "meaningful way," improvement has been minimal because the focus has been solely on using the EMR and not on learning how to integrate it effectively into the workflow of every business and clinical processes in a practice for the purpose of improving quality and efficiency.

Learn Your Software

From the moment computer technology first appeared on the front desks of medical practices, experts predicted that these efficient machines would eventually transform the cost and quality of healthcare in much the same way they had done for other industries. When quality improvement and cost-savings failed to materialize as fully as expected, these experts predicted that further gains would be achieved as computer processors became faster, storage capacity increased, and software became more sophisticated. This is comparable to saying that the efficiency of freeways would be improved if everyone drove a Ferrari, because each car would have the capability of traveling at faster speeds. Over time, speed, capacity, and software capabilities have all improved dramatically, but even with these "improvements," we have made little headway towards reaching the level of efficiency necessary for increasing the quality of healthcare and lowering its costs.

We rarely see a "non-computerized" practice today, and everyone, from the government on down, continues to believe that the inefficiencies in healthcare, which lead to high costs and low quality, will be "fixed" by the appropriate utilization of this technology. Significantly, current strategy includes an electronic health record; in fact, the utilization of an EMR is expected to become mandatory.

Healthcare analysts furthermore believe that in order for technology to have the greatest impact on cost and quality, physicians must practice in larger groups. This may all sound "easy;" yet, neither the implementation of new technology nor the process of merging practices always goes smoothly. One thing that has not changed in the past twenty years is that the single most consistent point-of-failure hindering achievement of these hoped for efficiencies lies at the doctor-technology interface, and the larger the group, the more exaggerated this bottleneck becomes. Since most processes flow through this interface, addressing this point-of-failure is essential to improving the cost and quality of healthcare and the profitability of group practices.

It is helpful to refer back to the time when technology was first being introduced into the healthcare industry in order to understand why new software can be difficult to implement. At that time, I visited the office of a friend who practiced in a busy group. He had computerized his practice a few years earlier, and I was anxious to evaluate the capabilities of his software. This doctor told me that I would have to speak with his staff about the software because he had no idea how to use it. This was at a time when the selection of software and the training necessary for its proper use were considered staff responsibilities. Since electronic medical records had yet to be fully developed, technology was being used primarily in the business and reception areas of a practice and served little to no clinical function. Physician involvement was considered unessential. In spite of the many subsequent developments in software, including sophisticated electronic medical records (which *do* impact the clinical aspects of a practice), most doctors still employ a "delegate to staff" attitude. Physicians often learn just enough about their software to "get by," which accounts for the fact that only a small percentage of them use the electronic medical records purchased by their groups in an effective manner, making it unlikely that these groups will capture the many efficiencies to be gained from sophisticated (and sometimes expensive) technologies.

It makes sense for all physicians to take the time to learn every essential feature of their software – features that will help them work more effectively, at the point of care, and also create greater efficiencies. This process will lead to reduced costs and increased revenue. It is the doctors who provide the money for purchasing new technology, and they are the ones who have the most to gain from its successful implementation. Because of this, they are the ones who should be most actively involved throughout the entire process.

Another problem with software implementation mentioned earlier is that most software companies are still anchored in an old sales style, one that primarily involves the physicians' staff. They are not accustomed to working directly with doctors, and are, perhaps, a little intimidated by them. Because of this, trainers from software companies request little of the doctors' time. In most cases, it is easiest for trainers to first implement the software functions for urgent billing and management needs (more front office focused) and put the electronic medical record implementation off until "later."

I feel that practitioners will achieve a more significant return from the investment they make in software when they understand that the greatest portion of the purchase and implementation costs of their new technology is their own time. This investment of time, and not the dollar amount of the purchase, is what is necessary for achieving long-term success. If physicians are not prepared to put in the time necessary for success, their return is unlikely to be worth the investment. It is not critical that they select the "best software on the planet"; rather, the success of a technology project is most dependent on the level of the user-physician's commitment to the project. It is important to realize too that the individual success of each doctor in a group is dependent upon his/her partners' levels of commitment as well as his/her own. Focusing on commitment at this single point-of-failure, before continuing to the next step, will give the greatest assurance that whatever software is chosen, whatever the costs, and however many problems are encountered along the way, the end results will be well worth the time and effort expended.

Efficient Data Entry

It is important to recognize that an EMR is but one component of an integrated software system, a system designed to improve total practice performance in much the same way that a carburetor is only one component of an integrated system designed to improve the overall performance of an automobile. The carburetor accounts for a percentage of an automobile's total performance in much the same way that an EMR accounts for a percentage of a practice's total performance. Maximum performance is achieved from utilization of the total system, not just this one component. An EMR cannot be considered in isolation from the practice management software; the two must be fully integrated to work as one, seamless unit.

Early EMRs were often stand-alone products, which required that practices using them employ more than one database. Some practices actually still do this. Not only does this require entry into two systems, but the databases do not "talk with one another." This provides numerous opportunities for errors and for reports which are unacceptable because they do not "connect" costs with clinical care and outcomes. For many long-established software companies, the EMR is an afterthought, while some that offer only EMRs claim that their products integrate with "most" practice management software programs. The problem is that this type of integration requires writing an interface to "connect" the two programs, programs that are written and updated continuously by two independent companies, with neither company taking the full responsibility for assuring that integration at the practice level will work seamlessly.

To achieve successful results, systems must be seamlessly integrated, with clinical and financial data remaining connected. One criterion that I stress as being critical for achieving improved efficiency and productivity is that data should be captured only one time – at the moment it is created. When we examine standard "business office" processes, we realize that the majority of both clinical *and* financial data is "created" in treatment rooms. Charges are often captured on paper charge slips and records recorded on paper charts in treatment rooms. At this point, the charges and medical records are "connected," but once the doctor completes these documents, they leave the treatment room and pass separately through all subsequent processes. This information becomes "disconnected." When software is not fully integrated in an electronic process, these electronic documents too remain "disconnected".

All good EMR packages should be capable of automatically capturing diagnostic and billing codes – as well as charges – from clinical notes, prompting for modifiers, and passing these codes and charges seamlessly to the point of patient check-out for cash collection and to billing for electronic submission. Patient treatment and billing should remain connected throughout the entire process. While some EMR companies claim that there is no disadvantage to using an interface (rather than having an EMR which is fully integrated with practice management software), bits of data can "fall through the cracks" between two separate software programs, with resultant lost charges and other types of errors which may lead to sub-optimal results.

Use an EMR to Capture Charges

Doctors would be surprised to learn that most of them fail to capture a significant percentage of the charges for the services they provide. One of the reasons for this is that, rather than marking charges for each patient as they "go along," physicians often put this task off until later – sometimes much later – virtually guaranteeing that a percentage of billable charges will "fall through the cracks." This is where an electronic medical record that simultaneously "pulls" treatment codes and charges throughout the documentation process can add value; this capability increases the percentage of charges captured. Of course, optimum capture of charges will result only if the documentation itself is completed in a timely manner – ideally, before the doctor "moves on" to his/her next patient.

Additionally, most studies show that, as a group, doctors tend to be "under-coders." Some say they prefer to stay "under the radar" for fear of being targeted for an audit. Others simply do not know the coding rules, do not keep up with changes, or fail to take the time necessary to document everything they do for their patients (a necessity for justifying appropriate codes). The goal is neither to under-code nor to over-code, but to code correctly. This is what it takes to receive the appropriate reimbursement for the services provided to patients. Since the coding process begins with the doctor, at the point of care, when s/he marks the diagnosis and treatment, there are no excuses for "getting it wrong." This is a task that is under the doctor's complete control, and today's technology can literally put the information necessary for "getting this right" at the doctor's fingertips.

Nothing will make a more immediate, positive impact on a practice's revenue than an increase in the collection ratio. No practice collects 100% of what is possible, but some collect substantially below this mark. In addition to the importance of documenting treatment and marking charges in a timely manner as discussed above, the following policies will all increase collection ratios: checking eligibility prior to patient visits, avoiding data entry errors at check-in and when marking charges, expediting the billing cycle, and following up on all claims that are denied or that pay less than expected. Most practices, upon switching to electronic capture of charges at the point of care (whether utilizing an electronic medical record or an electronic superbill), realize an increase in their collection ratios of at least seven percent. Consider how much revenue this 7% would represent in your practice, and you can imagine how productive your time would be if it were spent making your entire billing process more efficient and error free.

Collect Patient Portions at the Point of Care

In 2007, third parties paid approximately 88% of patient treatment costs, with patients paying only 12%. In a report recently published by Celent, a Boston-based research and consulting firm, researchers predicted that by the year 2012, this patient portion of payment will grow to 30%. Expectations are that this trend will continue. According to the Celent report, this increase in the patient's portion of the payment is likely to have dire consequences on a practice's cash flow – especially if that practice is one which either 1) is not equipped with information technology capable of facilitating the collection of clinical and financial data at the point of care or 2) employs business processes which require that insurance companies be billed and their payment received before requesting any payment from patients. As you know, any change in a billing process presents risks as well as opportunities. Let us look at the potential impact that placing a greater burden of the healthcare payment on patients might have on today's typical practice.

According to collection agencies serving all industries, cash that is collected on the day of service is typically 99% collectable, while this percentage falls to 72% for anything collected 90 days beyond this date. Consider the case of a hypothetical medical practice in 2007 (*Table 7.1*). Assume that this practice had average annual collections of $350,000. One can estimate, according to statistics from that year, that of this practice's $350,000 in revenue, 12% ($42,000) was collected from patients and the remaining 82% ($308,000) from third parties. Assume too that this practice allowed statements for the patient portion of billings to be sent out only after third party payments were received – typically around 90 days following treatment – and thus, fell into the category of which only 72% of the patient's portion of charges are typically collected. Further assume that the overhead of this practice was $210,000. These assumptions result in a predicted net income of $140,000.

Table 7.1: 2007 Practice Collecting 72% of Patient Portions

Payments from Patients (12%)	$42,000
Payments from Third Parties (82%)	$308,000
Total Payments	**$350,000**
Overhead	**$210,000**
Net Income	**$140,000**

Table 7.2 shows the potential drop in income for this same practice in the future year of 2012 – the date by which the Celent study has predicted that patients will be responsible for 30% of their charges. The doctor is still expecting to collect $350,000. The result, however, of this shift in payment responsibility is that our example practice's total patient portion of collections will increase from $42,000 to $105,000 (30% * $350,000 = $105,000), and the portion paid by third parties will decrease from $308,000 to $245,000 (70% * $350,000 = $245,000). This increase in patient responsibility for payments necessitates that our practice have an effective cash collection process in place. Assume, however, that as in our first scenario, this practice is still collecting only 72% of the patient portion of billings because it continues to initiate patient collections at a date far removed from the treatment date – 90 days following treatment. This results in only $75,600 of the expected $105,000 in patient charges being collected ($105,000 * 72% = $75,600). The result is that total collections would now be

$320,600, which is $29,400 less than the expected $350,000, and net income would drop by this amount (140,000 - $110,600 = $29,400).

Table 7.2: 2012 Practice Collecting 72% of Patient Portions

Expected Total Payments	$350,000
Expected Payments from Patients (30% of $350,000)	$105,000
Payments from Third Parties (70%)	$245,000
Actual Payments from Patients (72% of $105,000)	$75,600
Actual Total Payments	$320,600
Overhead	$210,000
Net Income	$110,600

The numbers in *Table 7.2* demonstrate the reduction in practice income that is likely to result from a shift towards greater patient responsibility for payment – especially for a practice that maintains a policy of billing patients at a much later date – only after insurance companies have been billed and their responses received.

A practice can take steps to avert this outcome, which is likely to come about as a result of the future expected shift in payment responsibility. For example, if our sample practice were to collect each patient's portion of his/her payment on the day of service, rather than waiting 90 days for billing, it is highly probable that more than 72% of these charges would be collected. Theoretically, by initiating a policy of same-day patient collections, the practice could collect 99% of the expected $105,000 in direct patient charges.

It is essential that practices take proactive steps such as this to avoid large declines in income as a result of the predicted future shift in payment responsibility. We have demonstrated how collection of patient portions on the date of treatment can be facilitated through effective employment of point-of-care technology. It can actually help us to accomplish even more.

We know from experience that when clinical and financial data are captured at the point-of-care and made immediately available at patient check out, the result, in addition to higher cash payments from patients, is a higher collection percentage of third party payments. To achieve this goal, we need the capabilities offered by an electronic medical record that is fully integrated with practice management software. In addition to collecting 99% of the patient's portion of charges, as in our example above, using point-of-care technology has been shown to increase third party collection ratios by at least 7%. This result is obtained because effective software captures all billable charges, reduces errors, codes correctly, and shortens the billing cycle.

Assume that our $350,000 example practice had been collecting 40% of its third party charges. We can work backwards to determine that this practice's total third party charges would have been $612,500 ($245,000 ÷ 40% = $612,500). If the practice were to collect an additional 7% of these charges through the use of effective technology, it would, theoretically, increase its third party collections by $42,875 ($612,500 ∗ 7% = $42,875). Note that this does not even take into account the ways in which such technology is anticipated to increase revenue in the future – through means such as documenting outcomes and thereby facilitating participation in "pay for quality" initiatives. As we move forward, keep in mind that future income will be significantly impacted by the effectiveness with which our practices adapt to this changing healthcare environment in which "quality" will be rewarded and patients will be responsible for a greater portion of payments. We need to prepare for this adaptation now.

Secure Your Medical Records

Because both doctors and patients have always considered medical documentation to be private information, doctors have always had to deal with security issues. With new technology and regulations (HIPAA), security issues have gained more attention and are becoming ever more complex. There is abundant supportive information to help a practice with HIPAA compliance, but before sifting through it all and planning your strategy, it is helpful to have a general understanding of the "economics of security." Armed with this knowledge, you will be better prepared for developing a security plan that will make economic "sense" for your practice.

All economic decisions involve tradeoffs. The issue of security presents a tradeoff between the actual cost of protection and the potential cost (or financial loss) should a security breach occur. At each extreme – either "no" security or "total" security – the economic costs are too high. It is easy to visualize the cost of "no" security. This is akin to practicing without malpractice insurance. At the other extreme, many doctors believe that "total" security is possible, or even affordable, because of technological innovations.

To better understand the economics of security, it helps to look outside the healthcare arena. For example, our local, state, and national governments endeavor to protect us from violent crime. Governments conduct cost-benefit analyses to determine how much to spend on a police force. We know that the more police on the street, the lower the crime rate. We also know that, beyond a certain point, the cost of putting more police on the street will exceed the benefit gained in terms of the degree of crime reduction.

In addition, we recognize that an "extreme" police presence in our communities might create unacceptable tradeoffs in terms of our individual freedoms and rights. We endeavor to seek an optimum balance between economics and security; society is willing to tolerate a certain amount of crime because we perceive that the benefit of attempting to reduce crime to zero is too costly, both in terms of money and our individual freedoms. As we approach medical security issues, we too need to find an optimum balance between value and cost.

HIPAA regulations are forcing doctors to take a second look at issues involving medical records security. I am often asked to compare the security of an electronic medical record with that of a paper one. Many doctors avoid electronic records, fearing that they will not be secure. They envision losses due to "electronic glitches" and feel that it might be too easy for information to fall into the wrong hands. Doctors seem to want a guarantee that electronic medical records will be 100% secure. What is amazing is how often these same doctors do not recognize the vulnerability of their paper records; they can be lost, stolen, or even totally destroyed in a fire or flood. Doctors seldom question the security of sending paper records through the mail or faxing them. They also leave them sitting on counters and allow unrestricted access by staff, even part-time filing clerks; yet, these same doctors are not confident about security when records are in a digital format that can be duplicated easily and stored in multiple locations (to prevent loss due to natural disasters or technology "glitches"), require security codes allowing only select employees to view specific sections of the record on a "need to access basis," and are transmitted in an encrypted format. All of these features clearly make the electronic record more secure than a paper one.

The economics associated with the security of medical records are no different than the economics for other security issues. Nothing can be 100% secured. If a hacker is determined to break into a system, s/he may find a way; however, the benefit derived from breaking into the records of a medical practice is not quite the same as, say, for entering the likes of the Bank of America or the CIA. Correspondingly, our budgets for firewalls and encryption do not need to be as great as those of these larger entities. Rules of common sense, and even HIPAA regulations, recognize this. If a security breach occurs, experience has shown that it is most likely to be low tech, such as a situation in which a doctor prints out a medical record and leaves it lying on a counter in public view, and this same thing happens regularly with paper records. Every security measure is vulnerable to this factor of "human error." The question to ask is, "Are electronic records substantially more secure than paper?" I think the answer, clearly, is, "yes!" We can achieve security in our practices in an economically feasible way, one in which the benefits substantially outweigh the costs.

Future Importance of the EMR

Even after a physician has chosen the "right" product for his/her practice, has successfully "gone live," and changed workflow to improve quality, efficiency, and productivity, the implementation process is not yet complete. The next step is to utilize the stored clinical data captured by the EMR for measuring patient outcomes, eliminating ineffective care, reducing treatment errors and omissions of recommended treatment, tracking follow-up care (to improve patient compliance), preventing disease and complications of disease, and participating in pay for performance and other quality initiatives designed to reward physicians for preventing disease and achieving better patient outcomes. To accomplish this, an EMR must employ specific treatment guidelines, and data must be stored in discrete, searchable fields.

PricewaterhouseCoopers (PWC) published a comprehensive research report several years ago entitled *HealthCast 2010* which covered trends and forces within the healthcare industry. Input for this report came from many of PWC's four thousand healthcare clients (including providers, health insurers, entitlements, employers, and service suppliers), along with input from 380 healthcare "thought leaders." One significant topic addressed in this report was the necessity of using treatment guidelines for reducing medical costs and improving quality. In the following statement, the report articulated the barriers that make it difficult to pursue this goal: "Medical professionals need to work toward global standards of medical treatment. In the United States, no national processes exist for developing standards of care."

While EMRs all come with a set of general medical guidelines, and some even come with a set of specialty-specific ones, these must be modified to fit each individual practice. This is something that must be done at the practice level and requires collaboration amongst the software company representatives, the physicians, and all staff members involved. All guidelines must be "hardwired" to correct codes, modifiers, and charges – which is easier for large groups that have management staff and can assign a few doctors to work with management. Smaller groups will need a strategy for attaining affordable help from their software companies, and they will need to collaborate with peers and share data in order to successfully employ evidence based medicine and participate in "pay for quality" initiatives.

Since most doctors do not yet have EMRs and clinical guidelines for measuring outcomes in place, quality initiatives such as pay for performance are currently based on claims, rather than outcomes, data. For example, if a company wants to provide an incentive for doctors to discuss smoking cessation with patients, all the payer can measure is whether or not the doctor discusses smoking cessation. One doctor may utilize a detailed guideline and spend several extra minutes discussing cessation with each patient while another might simply check a superbill, indicating that "smoking cessation" was discussed. Data from an EMR, however, might show that the doctor utilizing guidelines achieves a 40% cessation rate, while the other achieves only 5%. This would make it clear that the first doctor deserves a higher payment because, over the long term, this doctor's patients will be healthier, with resultant lower healthcare costs.

As mentioned earlier, the primary barrier to every initiative directed at improving the cost and quality of our healthcare system is located at the doctor-patient-technology interface. This is something that would change quickly if a critical mass of physicians were to actively embrace EMR technology and utilize it to its maximum capability. EMR technology capable of improving practice performance and positioning practices for evidence based medicine and the future of healthcare is available today. The challenge is to find a program and software company that are right for your practice, involve your doctors, develop a plan (in conjunction with an implementation team that can achieve your goals), and collaborate with peers in developing and testing clinical guidelines which can be shown to prevent disease and improve patient outcomes. This approach will greatly improve your chances of successful EMR implementation, and as successful implementations grow in number, the overall cost and quality of our healthcare system will continue to improve.

Reduce Errors with an EMR

The medical community can look to other industries when approaching the task of error reduction. Relatively few of the error prevention concepts proven long ago by other industries have been fully accepted by the healthcare industry and adapted to our delivery processes. A major barrier to initiating a process for reducing errors in medicine is our lack of recognition that individuals are not directly at fault for the vast majority of errors. Instead, as other industries have discovered, most errors result from "system failures," which, in turn, result from poorly designed processes. Taking a cue from industries that have successfully reduced their error rates, doctors must focus on error reduction through examination and improvement of the processes they utilize to connect the various steps in their patients' care as well as the communication processes throughout their practices and the facilities to which they refer patients.

The starting point in this process is recognition of the fact that error rates have little to do with either lack of intelligence or physician training and that fixing blame will only serve to worsen a problem. A comparison to the airline industry can give us deeper insight into this issue and offer possible solutions. The airlines are part of an industry in which, like medicine, relatively "small," easy to avoid errors can result in catastrophe. Let us start with what would seem to be an easily avoidable pilot error – somewhat equivalent to a doctor operating on the wrong body part. On takeoff, pilots (who are thoroughly trained) must extend flaps and slats on the plane's wings to add lift. If this step is omitted, the result can be fatal. Data shows that from the year 2000 to the 2009, pilots reported 55 cases in which they attempted to take off without properly extending these flaps. This seemingly "small," easy to make, error could have resulted in many fatalities. Fortunately, however, the airline industry had installed warning horns to alert pilots when they committed this oversight, and in all cases, these horns functioned properly, alerting pilots in time to avoid disaster.

Fortunately, the airline industry has not only implemented such processes, but has also adopted the policy of attaching no stigma to such incidents, making pilots unafraid to report them. They understand that the more data collected when these incidents occur, the more likely it is that safeguards will be found which will reduce their numbers in the future. According to Ben Berman, a former National Transportation Safety Board investigator, "You'll do the same thing correctly one million times and then not do it correctly one time. Things like a moment of stress, a spike in workload, a change in routine – all these things throw humans off track." As a matter of fact, distractions were found to be a factor in fatalities in Detroit and Dallas when flaps and slats were not deployed at takeoff.

Terry McVenes, an airline accident investigator, stated, "It's a good reminder for crews to understand that you've got to be following your procedures, and if there are interruptions while you are doing your checklists, you've got to stop and be vigilant to make sure you don't miss anything." His statement leads me to wonder what kinds of procedures and checklists medical professionals employ and how thoroughly they follow them, especially during busy or stressful times when interruptions are frequent. These preventative procedures and checklists are something we should adapt to our practices to lower error rates since they have already been proven to substantially reduce errors in other industries.

There are obvious parallels between the environment in which physicians practice and that in which commercial pilots fly. Clearly, stress, spikes in the workload, changes in routine, and distractions are normal occurrences in the typical day of both; however, unlike airline pilots, physicians have yet to embrace step-by-step procedures and checklists, and few "warning horns" exist for alerting doctors when steps in their treatment processes are omitted or performed incorrectly. Step-by-step guidelines do exist in healthcare, but they often are not implemented or diligently followed. The ease of use and effectiveness of clinical guidelines, which function much like a "checklist," can be greatly enhanced through the use of new electronic medical record technologies which offer the opportunity to enact the equivalent of "warning horns" when potentially harmful errors or omissions are made. If every physician were to actively utilize well thought out guidelines and incorporate them into his/her software, error rates could be drastically reduced, and treatment outcomes greatly improved, just as they have been in the airline industry.

Medicine is both an art and a science, and doctors tend to err on the side of "art," often resisting anything that might appear to be "cookbook medicine." While most believe that they consistently provide the care recommended by their specialty societies for specific conditions, a Rand study has shown that, on average, physicians fail to provide the recommend care 50% of the time. The reliance on "art and memory," rather than adhering to recommended clinical guidelines, increases the opportunity for errors and omissions – especially on "busy" days. When clinical guidelines are automated by electronic medical records, the opportunity for errors and omissions is greatly reduced because the doctor is prompted to consider all recommended exams, tests, treatments, and medications for each patient and condition. Follow-up does not "fall through the cracks." A recommendation will not be omitted as the result of "forgetting" because the use of automated guidelines will assure that the doctor consider all recommendations. Any omission is intentional, based on the doctor's consideration that a particular recommendation is unnecessary for a specific patient. This is where the "art" of medicine comes into play; the physician is using his/her experience and judgment to "make the call."

One of the most common sources of serious medical errors is prescribing the wrong medication. This error typically results from: prescribing an incorrect dosage, illegible handwriting, or overlooking a potential allergy or drug interaction. Electronic prescriptions can help to eliminate these errors as long as medication and allergy lists are kept current. Electronic prescription software can provide the equivalent of an airplane's "warning horn" and such software has been shown to reduce the number of such errors by 81%.

For example, as previously mentioned, an electronic prescription system can alert the doctor to an allergy or potential interaction at the moment a prescription is being "written." Although every doctor would agree that allergies and drug interactions are essential parts of the procedural "check list" which they should follow meticulously during the prescription writing process, they are sometimes missed. Most doctors believe they can do without written guidelines and check lists, backed up by electronic warnings, but they have been proven wrong. The number of errors being reported seems to be growing and this issue continues to make headlines. Electronic reminders will reduce errors – especially during hectic or stressful times. This "science" can enhance our art. Using technical "assistance" does not lessen our ability to apply the healing "arts" in practice; it simply enhances our treatment.

Reducing Treatment Variation with an EMR

It has been well documented that patients who have the exact same symptoms, clinical findings, and diagnoses receive a wide range of treatments. When Medicare analyzed 180,000 heart-attack patients in 1999, it was found that, "The quality of care provided heart-attack patients has more to do with their zip codes than with their medical condition. There is a wide gap between what we know and what we do." Many years ago, even the despised managed care organizations correctly identify "treatment variation" and "lack of physician follow-up" as two critical deficiencies within the healthcare delivery system – deficiencies that result in significantly higher costs, sub-optimal outcomes, and avoidable medical errors. Doctors are the only members of the healthcare community who can "fix" these deficiencies, but in addition to being a fragmented and independent group, doctors lack the time, resources, expertise, and central management capabilities required to coordinate a project of this scope and complexity.

A study conducted by Medstat in September 1999, found that only 29% of its sixteen thousand patients diagnosed with diabetes received the recommended annual eye exams, only 49% of the 3,949 patients with heart failure received an echocardiogram within three months of their initial diagnoses, and only 25% of the 6,404 asthma patients received the recommended anti-inflammatory drugs. The study found similar shortcomings in the recommended practice for patients with otitis media, low back pain, peptic ulcers, breast cancer, hypertension, and systemic heart disease. In the typical medical practice, no efficient mechanisms exist for: 1) measuring and comparing outcomes for any recommended course of treatment, 2) assuring that doctors follow-up, or 3) determining whether patients comply with instructions.

Medstat's findings were supported by United Healthcare's findings from an audit of its doctors in the early nineties which found that only 37% followed the American College of Cardiology's recommendation for beta blockers following a heart attack (for the purpose of avoiding a second attack), and only 59% of diabetic patients received the recommended annual glycated hemoglobin test. United also found that its doctors had no system for reminding patients about tests or reminding themselves to check whether or not patients were taking certain medications. Medstat found that even with overwhelming clinical evidence supporting certain treatment pathways, these often were not followed.

Quality is measured in all industries by the degree of variation from a desired standard. By this definition, quality in the healthcare industry will be improved and costs lowered when treatment variation is reduced. Unfortunately, the majority of physicians are independent, practice solo or in groups of five or fewer physicians, and have no incentive or mechanism for collaborating on solving this problem on a national scale; yet, until doctors begin to make this issue a priority, no meaningful healthcare reform that is capable of optimizing the needs of payers, patients, and doctors will be forthcoming.

In spite of the fact that studies and healthcare groups recognize the need for clinical guidelines (for collecting outcomes and cost data that can lead to "best practices" and reduce treatment variation), simply writing guidelines on paper and making them available to doctors has not proven to be an effective approach. The sheer number and complexity of guidelines make them cumbersome and impractical to use in a paper format at the point of care, and the inability to produce outcomes data using "paper" guidelines makes their adoption difficult. There is currently no resultant data that would compel a physician to change the way s/he treats a specific problem. Treatments are constantly changing, doctors are busy seeing too many patients, guidelines in paper-based reference manuals are too unwieldy, things easily fall through the cracks, and busy doctors cannot be asked to spend additional time searching for "correct" pathways, entering redundant data, and performing ever more documentation.

What is capable of improving the quality of a practice – and its bottom-line too – is software that is integrated, properly implemented, and capable of storing clinical data in discrete, searchable data fields – enabling this data to be retrieved at a later date for analysis of treatment outcomes. The software and technology capable of accomplishing these goals exist today, and individual doctors and groups can achieve these goals by working together with others in their specialties. The resultant quality improvements would lower malpractice occurrences through new, more complete and legible records, the elimination of certain medical errors – such as prescribing medication for a patient to which s/he is allergic or which will interact adversely with other drugs that s/he is taking – and preventing critical patient follow-up from falling through the cracks. For theses reasons, the effective application of technology, coupled with its ability to enable coordinated care amongst all those involved in healthcare, is at the top of the "quality improvement" list of virtually everyone who has a stake in the healthcare delivery system.

Consider Hiring a Medical Scribe

The vast number of physicians transitioning from paper to electronic medical records has spawned a new healthcare job description: the medical scribe. This scribe typically shadows a doctor and enters his/her patients' examinations, treatment plans, and follow-up conversations directly into an EMR. The driving force behind this new job category is the long-standing physician complaint that using an EMR is complex and requires too much "doctor time." This, they say, decreases the practitioner's productivity – some claim by as much as 30%. A 30% drop in productivity is obviously unacceptable for any practice, and the use of a medical scribe is one possible solution to this problem. Even physicians who have not experienced decreases in productivity as a result of their using an EMR perceive medical scribes as a way of increasing productivity – especially in a busy practice.

Medical scribes were first employed in emergency rooms, beginning in the mid-nineties. ScribeAmerica, a company based in Lancaster, California which was launched by an emergency room physician in 2003, trains high-quality scribes. If the growth rate of a single company is any indication of demand for the type of services that company provides, it is significant that, in 2010, ScribeAmerica's client base grew 60%. Emergency departments were likely candidates for the use of scribes because they treat high volumes of patients, and they adopted EMRs early on. Many of these emergency room scribes are part-time college students planning careers in medicine and see this as a training opportunity. Full-time career staff working in your practice can be trained to perform this task. While some expect the use of scribes to decrease as younger, tech savvy doctors enter into medical practice, I disagree. I think the biggest force driving their use will be physicians who are extremely busy and see a scribe as a way of boosting treatment quality and productivity by offering them more time for patient treatment.

Before the advent of electronic medical records, doctors already spent too much "patient care" time writing in charts and dictating. The relative amount of time spent examining and treating an emergency room patient relative to that spent documenting that same visit can be significant. Loma Linda Hospital has estimated that its doctors spend about two minutes with an ER patient and then take four more to enter the information from that visit into a computer. This means that for a six-minute visit, EMR documentation "eats up" 67% of the doctor's "patient time" – making the decision to initiate the use of scribes in the emergency room a "no-brainer."

In a medical practice, the relative differential between the time spent interacting with a patient and that required to enter the patient's information into the EMR varies by specialty and is not as dramatic as it is for the typical emergency room visit; however, the busier a practice, the more significant the impact that even a few minutes of documentation time, per patient visit, can have on productivity. For example, at 200 patient visits a week, in a forty-hour week, the average time, per visit, is 12 minutes. If the average amount of time that this doctor spends entering the history, exam, treatment, tests, patient conversations, and other clinical information into the electronic medical record requires three minutes, these "few minutes" represent 25% of the doctor's productive time. Multiply this by the number of patients seen weekly, and you can see just how much it would be worth for the doctor to capture this additional time for patient care. While one cannot put an exact dollar amount on its value, it is likely that redirecting this documentation time to patient treatment would translate to an increase in productivity of a percentage approaching 25% of the practice's revenue. For a practice averaging 200 visits a week, the financial outcome could be substantial – a value that would easily be equivalent to many times the cost of the scribe.

While the opportunity to increase productivity is one good reason for a busy practitioner to consider the use of a medical scribe, given the expected direction of healthcare – where the intent is eventually to pay for quality, prevention, wellness, and coordinated care – all of which *require* the use of an EMR – the value of utilizing a scribe is likely to be even greater. When determining whether hiring a scribe would be beneficial for your practice, a good place to start your analysis would be to measure the percentage of your patient care time you currently utilize entering data into your electronic medical record. Assuming your average documentation time is three minutes, the chart below shows the percentage of your time spent documenting a patient visit based on a range of average visit times. If your average documentation time is higher, or lower, than three minutes, you can adjust the spreadsheet accordingly. If your documentation time exceeds 15% of your total patient care time, and you have a backlog of more than two days for seeing a non-urgent new patient, I feel that the use of a medical scribe is definitely worth investigating.

Table 7.4: Documentation Time as a Percentage of Dr's Time

Average Visit Time	Average Documentation Time	Documentation Time as a percentage of Dr's Total Time
5	3 Minutes	60.00%
10	3 Minutes	30.00%
15	3 Minutes	20.00%
20	3 Minutes	**15.00%**
25	3 Minutes	12.00%
30	3 Minutes	10.00%

Chapter 8

Increase the Size of Your Practice

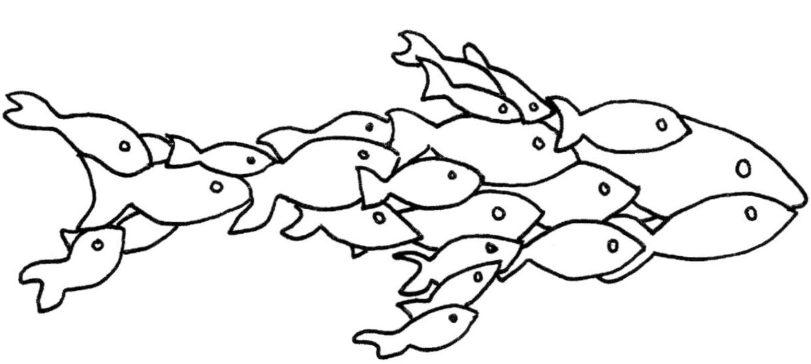

The More the Merrier: Profiting from the Group Model

If offered a 50% increase in income, would you turn down the opportunity – especially if this offer did not require you to work any harder than you do now, allowed you to take more time off, and enabled you to focus on the areas of practice that you most enjoy and for which you achieve your best outcomes? Even in medicine's current environment of high volume and low fees, all of these benefits can be achieved when three or more solo practices come together and implement a well-planned, well-executed practice merger.

In spite of the vast number of well-documented benefits that group practice can provide, many doctors still practice solo or in small groups. There are a myriad of long-term advantages and opportunities to be gained through practicing in a group, but aside from these long-term opportunities, a merger makes sense for the immediate economic advantages alone. Consider the instant benefits to be obtained through the creation of a group practice under one roof – say, a group formed through a merger of three physicians practicing solo in the same geographic area. For ease of comparison, assume that each of these practices has the same annual financial structure: $380,000 in revenue and $220,000 in overhead, resulting in $160,000 profit. Although the economics of newly merged practices are likely to improve in a number of areas, to keep this example simple, we will consider only two areas of potential savings – those generated through "sharing" the costs of rent and staff. A "typical" merger of three practices into a blended practice under one roof could easily capture the savings in rent and staff indicated in *Table 8.1*.

As a result of post-merger overhead savings, the combined profit for the practices represented in this table goes from $480,000 ($160,000 + $160,000 + $160,000 = $480,000) to $720,000 – a 50% increase! Note that the overhead ratio in this example drops from 57.9% to 36.8%. The result is that each doctor in the group is now able to keep $63.20 of each $100 collected, rather than $42.10, and this is accomplished without seeing any more patients than before the merger.

Table 8.1: A Three-Practice Merger

	Practice A	Practice B	Practice C	Post Merger
Revenue	$380,000	$380,000	$380,000	$1,140,000
Rent	$50,000	$50,000	$50,000	$87,000
Staff	$120,000	$120,000	$120,000	$183,000
Other expenses	$50,000	$50,000	$50,000	$150,000
Total Expenses	$220,000	$220,000	$220,000	$420,000
Profit	$160,000	$160,000	$160,000	$720,000
Overhead Ratio	57.9%	57.9%	57.9%	36.8%

The outcome for this example merger is achieved simply as a result of cost savings. Obviously, the results would be less dramatic had the pre-merger overhead ratios been lower. Conversely, for cases in which the pre-merger overhead ratios are higher, the increase in post-merger profit will be even greater. What is important to note is that if you are planning a merger, with the goal of increasing your profit margin, the foundation of your merger strategy must be the reduction of "unnecessary" overhead; otherwise, it is unlikely that the implementation plan you put in place will be capable of achieving this goal.

Once practices have merged, achieved efficient operations, and are producing higher profit ratios, additional opportunities "suddenly" arise. For one thing, the "new" practice is larger and more visible, which in itself stimulates growth. It is now easier to cover the office full-time – expanding patient access. Also, because doctors typically possess different skill sets, the practice can offer patients an expanded array of services. These changes increase patient satisfaction, stimulate growth, and allow each participating doctor to focus on the areas in which s/he excels. As we look to a future that will surely involve the employment of quality improvement, documentation of outcomes, and evidence based medicine, merged practices will also be better positioned for participating in pay for performance and other "pay for quality" incentives.

Doctors who choose not to merge practices with others often cite their reason for remaining in solo practice as the fear of losing autonomy in decision making. There is no question that some autonomy is lost once you are no longer the sole decision maker; yet, how much autonomy do doctors actually have in a healthcare market that is increasingly dominated by major employers, insurance companies, large medical groups, and the government? Besides, this small "loss" is more than offset by the resultant increase in cash flow and the enjoyment of practicing in an environment of camaraderie brought about by working with partners. Doctors who remain in solo practice are paying a high price for maintaining the right to be lone decision makers. In the example outlined above, a doctor choosing to remain solo would be giving up 50% of his or her potential income to overhead and would be poorly positioned to capture the future group practice opportunities projected by healthcare thought leaders. Since there is no specific limit to the number of practices that can merge into a single group, a three-practice merger might simply be the starting point.

Cutting Relative Costs by Merging

In an economic downturn, one of the first things managers of medical practices do is look for ways to cut costs. While, in good times as well as bad, it makes sense to cut *unnecessary* costs, it does not make sense to cut anything beyond "the fat" without first weighing all alternatives. There actually may not be much "fat" to cut because, ideally, a well-run business will be operating the same in both good and bad economies. A previously mentioned business axiom to consider before downsizing is the following: "You cannot cut your way into prosperity." What I like about this adage is that it encourages the consideration of strategies that go beyond simple cost-cutting. If overhead costs are way out of line, cost-cutting is definitely in order; however, if one's goal is prosperity (rather than simply maintaining profit over the short-term), a doctor should consider cutting "relative costs" rather than cutting into the "core" of his/her practice.

What I am referring to here as "relative", as opposed to "actual," costs are the average costs-per-patient as opposed to total practice costs. These costs-per-patient are the relevant ones to monitor. I use the term "relative" because the average cost-per-patient can be declining even as total costs increase. Let us take a look at a practice with the same statistics as the three practices in our previous merger example, with the additional information that each practice has 3,500 annual patient visits. Practices A, B, and C each have an average cost-per-patient of $62.86 ($380,000 ÷ 3,500). Post-merger, the new total costs for the group are $420,000, and patient volume has tripled to 10,500. Even though total costs have increased from $220,000 to $420,000, the average cost-per-patient has dropped from $62.86 to $40.00 ($420,000 ÷ 10,500). Also, as shown in the previous table, the overhead ratio declined from 57.9% for the individual practices, to 36.8% for the group. A decline in the average cost-per-patient and overhead ratio is typically seen with efficiency improvement, practice mergers, or when patient volume is growing. Merging two or more practices offers this type of opportunity for the merging practitioners – the opportunity to share the substantial costs of rent and staff salaries, and it opens the possibility of decreasing cost-per-patient and total overhead percentage dramatically while simultaneously increasing the doctors' compensations. Most importantly, the participating practices are prospering and still have their cores in tact for future growth.

Obviously, running a practice at a significantly lower cost-per-patient makes sense in any economic environment. As more doctors join a group, this cost-per-patient continues to drop (as long as proven efficiency principles are simultaneously employed), and new opportunities primarily available to group practices begin to open up. Given that many doctors practice solo or in groups of five or fewer, this opportunity to add doctors or merge practices is available to many, and it makes sense regardless of what type of healthcare reform is adopted in the future.

Leveraging Advantages Beyond Cost Reduction

Size influences the effectiveness of a medical practice in much the same way that it influences the effectiveness of any type of business. Each business "size" enjoys certain advantages and disadvantages in the marketplace. Traditionally, small businesses have less available capital, but are able to compensate for this disadvantage by being more flexible and offering more personalized service. They are able to make faster decisions and move more quickly on opportunities. Additionally, small businesses are often able to command a higher price for their personalized services. Traditionally, larger businesses have tended to move more slowly, but their greater access to capital has made it easier for them to invest in equipment and information technology, pay for more qualified employees, and spend more dollars on marketing and advertising services.

In the past, the best, large, high-volume businesses utilized improved business processes to achieve economies of scale and were thereby able to decrease costs while improving quality and offering a wider array of services. Today, innovative business processes, combined with the more effective use of information technology (which has become ever more affordable), is blurring the lines between large and small businesses – allowing larger businesses to maintain their traditional advantages while also capturing those available to smaller ones – quicker response and greater flexibility. These strategies can be applied effectively to medical practices.

Based on my experience working with practices of all sizes, doctors practicing in groups – especially those of five or more, well trained, hard working doctors – typically are able to leverage their group's efficiencies and earn substantially above the average incomes reported within their specialties. With improved business processes and greater efficiencies, I expect future group models to leverage their existing advantages even more – increasing their ability to profitably meet the needs of patients, payers, employers, and government agencies alike. This is possible because the advantages of being part of a large group go far beyond mere cost reduction, enabling profits to be increased in multiple ways. Following are some of the more significant advantages to be obtained through practicing in a group.

Increased Negotiating Clout

It is widely recognized that third party payers prefer to work with larger groups. It is more efficient for them to negotiate with entities representing a large number of providers; however, this advantage is offset if a group is unable to control quality at all practice locations, and this happens frequently. Effective quality management is especially difficult for IPAs and PPOs that are composed of independent practitioners who have come together *strictly* for the purpose of negotiating contracts. Larger groups will be more successful at negotiating better paying contracts if they integrate operations and electronic medical records, thereby enabling them to measure quality of care, set benchmarks, and manage more effectively. Because delivering better quality translates to improved outcomes for patients – with accompanying savings for third party payers – these larger groups will be able to secure improved contracts; under "pay for performance" guidelines, they will be rewarded because they will be delivering greater value. These effective groups will also be achieving higher patient satisfaction – a critical factor for future success when re-negotiating contracts. Groups with lower patient satisfaction ratings will be willing to settle for less. Larger groups also enjoy similar negotiating clout when meeting with vendors to set the price and terms for industry products and/or services the group seeks to purchase.

Gains from Group Efficiency

Typically, the larger an entity, the greater its opportunity for leveraging the benefits associated with improvements in efficiency. In the past, many businesses said that they were achieving "economies of scale" when they improved their efficiency – something mostly focused on reducing the per-unit cost of production. With the use and integration of quality management tools and today's technology, doctors achieve efficiencies in their practices and are able to simultaneously improve both the quality of treatment and practice productivity, while lowering costs. The challenge lies in recognizing that efficiency improvement does not occur automatically just because a group is large; achieving greater efficiency and quality requires a strong commitment to rigid adherence to scientific principles on the part of the individual physicians within the group.

Medical practices can capture additional advantages through the formation of large groups because they are classic examples of the "high fixed cost" economic model. Their high fixed costs are the key to capturing these advantages. Costs considered "fixed" are those discussed in Chapter One – those that are unaffected by increases or decreases in volume and remain constant, no matter how "busy" a practice is – and these costs are high in a medical practice. Efficiencies implemented in the form of improved throughput enable the large volume of a group practice to be spread over existing fixed costs, providing an advantage over small group or solo practitioner models with their lesser volumes. As a practice increases patient volume and/or the number of services it provides, the majority of its costs remain constant, creating the opportunity to capture, as profit, a large portion of the additional revenue produced. The net effect is that, if fixed costs are not raised, the greater the volume of services, the more the overhead percentage drops – resulting in higher profit margins for all group members.

Offering a Wider Array of Services Improves Customer Satisfaction

A large group can offer a wider array of services than a smaller one. No physician is interested in every aspect of his/her specialty, and no one is good at everything. A group offers individual doctors the opportunity to focus on the areas they most enjoy and at which they are most skilled. Each doctor brings his/her particular skills to a single or multi-specialty group and creates a new resource for referrals in his/her area of specialization, sub-specialization, or special interest. Large practices are in an enhanced position to attract new associates who have unique skills, and they can more easily subsidize these associates' salaries through the transition period required for them to build their own referrals and become capable of financially supporting both their salaries and the overhead that they generate. If a practice is lacking in a specific service or area of interest, there is opportunity for growth in that area. For single specialty practices, this could include bringing in practitioners from other specialties to offer medical or surgical services in areas complimentary to their practices.

A complete array of services makes a group practice a "one stop shop," with experts who are able to handle any type of condition that might be presented. This is not only attractive to patients but also leverages the group's marketing and contract negotiating opportunities. Also, the ability to collaborate with peers within the group – to obtain quick second opinions from practitioners with specific expertise pertinent to difficult cases – is something that makes practice more enjoyable for the doctors within the group and offers incalculable benefit to patients.

Increased Patient Access

Inability to gain quick access to a practice is one of the most common patient complaints and has accounted for the failure of many HMOs. A well-managed, large, group practice is able to provide quick access because it can offer an alternate doctor who is not fully booked when the patient's "regular" doctor is unavailable. For example, when a member doctor is out on vacation, or is away attending a seminar, his/her patients can still be appointed, with no backlog building while s/he is gone. Multi-location groups provide the additional convenience of nearby locales.

Large groups are also able to expand capacity and improve access even further because they have the personnel to cover part-time, off-site, and specialty clinics. Specific conditions or patient types can be handled more efficiently in specialized "venues" in which patients with similar conditions are seen in large numbers at one location. All of these advantages enable quicker access, allowing patients to be seen at the time they are most motivated, and this leads to practice growth. This easy access, which is enabled by the large group model, offers a strategic advantage that is difficult for small groups to duplicate.

Groups Have Greater Access to Capital

Many opportunities require a capital investment in space and/or equipment, and in this area, groups have always had an advantage. A group's larger number of practitioners and more sizable lines of credit provide them with more immediate access to capital. This enables them to grow, increase space, add locations, invest in equipment, and move quickly on new opportunities. Initially, physician practice management companies that purchased practices and formed large groups justified the need for their services with the promise that they would invest in the sophisticated information technology necessary for a group to collaborate and capture group efficiencies; however, it often happened that they did not follow through on these promises. With today's lower prices for sophisticated information technology, group practices can now, themselves, afford to invest in and fully implement the information systems crucial to the success of their practices.

Groups Have Greater Opportunity to Add Ancillary Income

While all companies have multiple sources of revenue, these sources are not equally profitable. In competitive industries, the core business of many companies is typically the least profitable revenue source (sound familiar?). Consider the automobile industry of the past. There are many sources of profit in the auto industry, but the highest profits are not always generated from activities that produce the highest revenues (such as manufacturing and distribution). Ford is in the auto manufacturing business; yet, at one point in history, almost 50% of the company's profits were generated from financing! Considering that financing only accounted for 20% of Ford's total revenue, one might wonder what business Ford was really in at that time. The important lesson physicians can learn from this is that Ford was able to capture the higher profit margins associated with auto financing only because the company was in the auto manufacturing and distribution business in the first place.

A competitive model relevant to physician groups is U-Haul. Physicians can learn much by studying U-Haul's strategy within the U.S. consumer truck-rental business. According to a paper published in *Harvard Business Review* by Orit Gadish and James L. Gilbert, U-Haul, Ryder, Hertz-Penske, and Budget waged a battle for market share in the early 1990s. U-Haul was considered to be at a disadvantage because it charged the lowest prices and had the oldest fleet of trucks; however, in spite of the fact that it barely broke even on its rental business, U-Haul was the most profitable company in the industry – and by a wide margin. The industry's average operating margin was less than 3%; yet, U-Haul's was 10%!

As in the Ford example, U-Haul's greatest source of profit was not its core business – truck rental. U-Haul understood something about the business that its competitors had missed. According to the authors of the *Harvard Business Review* piece, "All the ancillary products and services consumers need to complete the job has only begun when they rent a truck." When consumers rent a truck, they need ancillary products and services such as boxes, insurance, trailers, and storage space. While margins in the truck rental business are low because consumers shop for the best rates, those in the ancillary business are high. In order to gain this ancillary business, however, one must first capture the "parent" truck-rental business. Similarly, Ford had to be in the auto business in order to profit from auto "accessories."

A physician's core business is patient care, but higher margins are potentially available in healthcare-related ancillaries – especially those that have synergies with that core business. As in the examples of U-Haul and Ford, physicians can pursue these higher margin, ancillary businesses because they are already in the business of healthcare delivery. They must be aware, however, that not all ancillaries are equally profitable for each specialty, especially if they are not synergistic with the core business.

While early attempts at organizing physicians into networks and "companies" met with mixed success, it is becoming clear that there are higher margin, ancillary healthcare services which have synergies with certain specialties. Relevant specialty groups can manage these services best, and at lowest cost. Physicians are typically focused on those ancillaries with the highest revenues but it is important to note that these are not necessarily the ones with the highest profits. There will be many ancillary opportunities available to physicians in group practices because these groups can offer efficiencies. It is important that these groups examine all the possibilities open to them and seek the ancillaries that are most synergistic with their specialties. While ancillaries have the potential of adding profitability for the physician, they also create value for the payer and better service for the patient – creating true win-win-win situations.

A multitude of ancillary opportunities exist in many specialties, but because of their requirements in terms of cost and patient volume, it is difficult for a one or two-doctor practice to participate in these opportunities. Groups are better able to absorb the financial risks involved in developing sources of ancillary income (such as ambulatory surgery centers or physical therapy services) and in purchasing income producing diagnostic equipment (such as MRI or ultrasound). Most ancillary services have high fixed costs, as do medical practices, making them dependent on volume for success. Groups typically have the volume necessary for reducing this financial risk associated with ventures dependent on size and can provide these ancillary services more efficiently, making them more cost effective.

Larger Groups Are More Visible than Smaller Ones

Larger groups have a significant marketing advantage. This is due in part to three factors: enhanced visibility, the opportunity to pool resources for the purposes of PR and advertising, and the ability to leverage individual physicians' reputations in the community. Larger groups, whether at single or multiple locations, attract more attention because of their increased visibility. In addition to visibility, pooling advertising dollars offers a significant advantage. For example, a solo practitioner might invest $15,000 a year in marketing, which accomplishes very little. Investing this same amount, per doctor, provides a fifteen-doctor group with a $225,000 marketing budget – one that can produce wide exposure through various types of media. Generally, too, if some doctors within a group are well known and enjoy good reputations in the community, their reputations are "transferred" to the other doctors in the group – a significant advantage, especially for new practitioners.

A Group Can Designate a Managing Partner

Many doctors are either unskilled at business management or do not enjoy it. They prefer to practice medicine exclusively yet are often faced with the responsibility for duties related to business management. This presents a hardship for many practitioners. Of necessity, doctors practicing solo must be competent business managers if their practices are to survive. Group practices often have at least one member doctor who has a specific interest in management and is accomplished at it. This benefits all doctors in the group. Larger practices can even afford to support the efforts of a managing partner by reducing his/her patient care hours, assisting him/her by hiring a full-time manager, and utilizing the services of consultants and advisors at times when specific types of expertise are needed (such as expertise in HR, compliance, coding, electronic medical record technology, or process improvement). This affords the doctors who are not as skilled at, or as interested in, management the opportunity to focus solely on patient care – a definite advantage for both them and their patients.

Lifestyle Benefits of the Group Practice

One significant reason many doctors choose to be part of a group is that they want benefits similar to those corporations can provide – benefits that enable them to have personal lives. These include: regular hours, paid vacations, call coverage, sick leave, health insurance, and retirement plans. As stated above, many doctors dislike the headaches and responsibility associated with management duties, and a group can have a managing partner or business manager who handles these benefits. A group practice can provide doctors with many of the same benefits that a large corporation provides its employees, yet, allow them to still maintain more control over their future than the typical corporate employee.

Another advantage of the group structure is that it provides an exit strategy for a doctor who is ready to retire. Because doctors in a group have the option of ownership, they may have a partnership interest that they can sell at retirement – something typically more difficult for doctors in smaller practices to accomplish. For practitioners in a two or three doctor practice, it is often a financial hardship for the remaining doctors to buy-out the ownership interest of a retiring partner; however, in a large group where a buy-out is spread over ten, twenty, or more doctors, the hardship for each individual member is greatly reduced. Also, even though the group may have a pension plan, it is an advantage for the retiring partner to be able to retain some of the equity s/he has built in practice over a long career. In addition to owning tangible assets, such as equipment and accounts receivable, the retiring doctor also owns an intangible asset in the form of the cash flow that s/he generates. This cash flow has a value, and it is more likely to continue at the same level in a group practice, making the "buy-out" of a retiring doctor more feasible.

Start Small: Adding an Associate Can Dramatically Improve Profit

Leaders in every business seek ways of improving their profit margins. For those in growth industries, or ones where there is little competition, improving the profit margin may simply be a matter of raising fees. With little effort and no change in business operations, the business becomes more profitable – virtually overnight; however, for those in price-competitive industries, improving the profit margin is not so simple. For most doctors, improving profit margins will require working harder, cutting costs, and expanding hours. While these options are always available, two more palatable options which have great potential for increasing profit, yet are utilized infrequently or implemented in ways that fail to capture much of their potential opportunity, are: adding an associate and/or merging with another practice. In order to better understand the economics of these opportunities and how one might capture the full potential from either of them, a doctor needs to understand the concept of marginal profit and focus on increasing it rather than gross profit.

When doctors focus on profit, they tend to look only at *gross profit* margins, leading them to make poor decisions regarding the implementation of productivity improvement strategies for increasing profit. If a practice's overhead is 65% of revenue, the gross profit margin on what it collects is 35%. Most doctors are well aware of this gross profit margin, often remarking that they (in this case) "keep only 35%" of what they collect. This can lead to complacency – the attitude of, "I can't afford to change. How can I afford to pay an associate more than 35% of his/her productivity, or merge with another practice, when my profit margin is only 35%?" This is a misconception, and it often results in unsuccessful negotiations with associates or in mergers that never get off the drawing board. The profit margin that actually results from seeing more patients (or providing more services) in this example practice with 65% overhead will not be 35%; in fact, it could as high as 85%!

Let us see how this can be accomplished, using an example of a solo practitioner whose overhead is 65% (*Table 8.2*). In this example, revenue is $392,000, expenses $254,785, and net profit $137,215. The gross profit margin is 35.00% ($137,215 ÷ $392,000 = 35.00%). In other words, this doctor keeps thirty-five cents of each dollar collected. While it is useful to know this gross profit margin, it is more important to be aware of the *marginal profit* that will be produced from any new revenue generated. This is the profit that a practice will generate from seeing patients who are not a part of its current volume. For this calculation, we need to know which costs will increase as volume increases and which will remain fixed. Of the expenses listed in *Table 8.2*, only three will increase along with volume: medical supplies, office supplies, and lab fees (the ones marked with asterisks). These three expense categories account for 14.35% of the total costs incurred by the practice at its current patient volume level (7.78% + 1.8% + 4.77% = 14.35%). Using this percentage, we can now estimate what the new expenses associated with additional volume will be, and this is 14.35% of any new revenue generated. This means that our profit margin for the additional revenue generated from each patient seen beyond our current volume is 85.65% (100% - 14.35% = 85.65%) – not 35.0%.

Table 8.2: Example Practice Financial Statement

Revenue		% of Total
Fees	$380,000	96.94%
Supply Sales	$12,000	3.06%
Total Revenue	**$392,000**	**100%**
Expenses		
Advertising	$1,800	0.71%
Computers	$5,600	2.20%
Dues & Subscriptions	$2,900	1.14%
Donations	$700	0.27%
Equipment lease	$1,500	0.59%
Entertainment	$350	0.14%
Insurance (health)	$12,500	4.91%
Insurance (Malpractice)	$7,300	2.87%
Insurance (Work comp)	$2,200	0.86%
Interest expense	$4,200	1.65%
Janitorial	$4,935	1.94%
Legal & Accounting	$1,800	0.71%
* Medical Supplies	$19,820	7.78%
Meetings CME	$1,680	0.66%
* Office Supplies	$4,580	1.80%
* Lab	$12,160	4.77%
Postage	$3,120	1.22%
Rent	$34,000	13.34%
Payroll	$118,000	46.31%
Storage	$3,240	1.27%
Telephone	$8,600	3.38%
Utilities	$3,800	1.49%
Total Expenses	**$254,785**	**100%**
Net	**$137,215**	
Overhead Ratio		**65.00%**
Gross Profit Margin		**35.00%**

If practice revenue were to increase by $50,000 in this example, the increase in costs associated with this revenue increase would be $7,375 ($50,000 * 14.75% = $7,375), not the $32,500 ($50,0000 * 65.0% = $32,500) that we would expect if we were to calculate costs using our original 35% gross profit margin. Treating these additional patients actually results in $42,625 in new profit ($50,000 – $7,375 = $42,625) – far more than the $17,500 ($50,000 - $32,500 = $17,500) we would have expected had we used the gross profit margin for figuring our profit rather than the marginal profit margin. Understanding this concept of marginal profit will dramatically change how a doctor approaches salary negotiations with associates or potential merger opportunities with other practitioners.

When negotiating mergers, associateships, or partnerships, focus is traditionally on the productivity of the individual doctors involved, often ignoring the profit margin benefit that will accrue to all of them if an affiliation is formed. As in the process of merging a practice, or when a doctor takes on an associate, the goal is to spread a greater volume of patients over relatively constant costs. This creates tremendous profit leverage. Obviously, efficient practice processes will be essential to keeping fixed expenses "fixed" until capacity is reached. When the need to increase fixed costs eventually arises (adding staff or space), this should be done with a focus on increasing productivity along with capacity (treating more patients and/or providing more services per hour). This will also have a leveraged effect on profit.

In the majority of cases, adding the "right" associate to a solo practice has the potential of doubling revenue in about five years. What is seldom recognized is that this doubling of revenue has a leveraged impact on profit; note that doubling revenue more than doubles profit. *Table 8.2* demonstrates this effect. In our previous practice example, the doctor is producing $392,000 annually, with 14.35% in marginal overhead costs, and taking home $137,215. If an associate were able to double this revenue figure in five years, the fifth year's revenue would be $784,000, but the cost increases associated with this new volume would be only $56,249 ($392,000 * 14.35% = $56,252), resulting in $335,748 additional profit to the practice ($392,000 - $56,252 = $335,748). This would increase total profit from $137,215 to $472,963 ($137,215 + $335,748 =

$472,963). The end result is that, while revenue increases 100%, profit increases 244.7%!

Table 8.2: Result of Associate "Efficiently" Doubling Revenue

	Before	After	$ Change	% Change
Revenue	$392,000	$784,000	$392,000	100.0%
Expenses	$254,785	$311,037	$56,252	22.1%
Profit	$137,215	$472,963	$335,748	244.7%

When we examine the opportunity in our example at the end of five years, we see that if both doctors were paid the exact same salary at this five year mark, each would make $236,481 a year. For the owner (who made a smart investment five years earlier), this income is approximately $100,000 a year more than he was receiving at his starting point five years ago – and he is receiving this without seeing any extra patients! If this doctor has a fifteen-year retirement horizon, this increase represents a future opportunity of $1,500,000 – and this is before considering any other opportunities that may be available to him in the next fifteen years (such as adding a third associate or increasing his and/or his new partner's productivity). It is important to note that, even if a practice increases fixed costs due to a need for more staff, the assumption is that this is being done with the purpose of increasing productivity by at least the amount of these new staff salaries. If so, this will not negatively impact profit.

When a solo or small group practice takes on a new associate, the challenge lies in determining how to avoid losing money in the first year, compensate the associate throughout the process, and eventually form a mutually equitable partnership. How do the doctors work it out so that the group stays together and the long-term value (in this example case, $1.5 million for the original owner) is captured? The primary barriers to establishing a successful associateship in a solo practice or small group are: 1) determining how to provide the associate with a fair salary and 2) determining an affordable "price" for the buy-in. This is when understanding profit margins and how they impact the transition period along the road to partnership is crucial.

From the perspective of the typical owner, in our example, the assumption is that because his/her gross profit margin is 35%, the associate must be paid less than 35% of his/her productivity. The owner feels that paying the associate above this level will cause the practice to lose profit, but the end result of paying a low percentage of productivity in the initial years of an associateship is the likelihood that the associate will not receive a livable wage. In reality, other than the risk of having to subsidize the associate's salary to a small extent in the first year, s/he can be paid above this overhead percentage, and far from losing money, the owner will make additional profit throughout this transition period. Let us see why this is the case.

For purposes of this example, I have suggested "reasonable" yearly salaries for an associate joining our sample solo practice – a case in which the owner perceives that there is insufficient cash flow to support the associate.

Table 8.3: Five-Year Financial Opportunity

	Associate's Productivity	Marginal Cost	Cost Increase	Associate Salary	Percent Compensation
Year One	$78,400	14.35%	$11,250	$67,150	86%
Year Two	$156,800	14.35%	$22,500	$95,000	61%
Year Three	$235,200	14.35%	$33,751	$120,000	51%
Year Four	$313,600	14.35%	$45,000	$140,000	45%
Year Five	$392,000	14.35%	$56,252	$160,000	41%
Total	$1,176,000	14.35%	$168,753	$582,150	50%

Assume that in the first year, the associate produces $78,400 in revenue and that s/he increases this production by the same amount each year, for four years, until, in the fifth year, s/he produces $392,000. The associate is paid $67,150 in year one, which is 86% of his/her productivity. At this salary, the owner breaks even. It is important to note that, typically, an associate will produce much better than this in the first year, allowing him/her to be paid more than in our example while providing the owner with a small profit.

Each year the associate's salary can be increased as his/her compensation, as a percentage of productivity, drops. In our example, at the end of five years, the associate's cumulative productivity has reached $1,176,000, and s/he has been compensated a total of $582,150 – averaging 50% of his/her productivity over the five years. Even with a pay level at 50% of productivity, and considering the accompanying increased costs to the practice of $168,748, the total cost of the associate to the owner over the five years would be $750,898 ($168,748 + $582,150 = $750,898), leaving $425,101 in additional profit from these five years for the owner ($1,176,000 - $750,898 = $425,102).

As mentioned earlier, the biggest stumbling blocks to capturing an opportunity such as this are reaching an agreement regarding the associate's salary and establishing the eventual buy-in process for becoming a partner. My recommendation is that the owner treat the first year's salary as an investment. Had the associate in this example been paid $87,150 in the first year – instead of $67,150 – when s/he was still producing only $78,400 (which is unlikely), the practice would have "lost" $20,000, but this would have been a small investment for the owner given the future upside potential of this relationship. The details of the buy-in process can create stumbling blocks. All associates are not equally productive; yet, in my experience, the opportunity to be captured from taking one on and retaining him/her over the long-term is usually even greater than what I have presented in this example.

While the impact that a new associate will have on a practice can vary substantially, especially by specialty or due to initial practice revenue, the fact that most of today's well-trained associates produce significantly higher figures than those used in this example leaves little to fear financially for a busy doctor in need of hiring one. Ideally, the associate will accrue buy-in credit while working towards partnership, and the amount accrued can be determined by the amount of profit captured by the owner-doctor throughout the transition process, coupled with the amount predicted to be generated going forward into the future as partners. In my experience, the amount of money an owner will make during the transition process and going forward into the future with the associate as a partner is substantially greater than 50% of the practice's "starting value." An owner doctor should base any associateship decisions on future opportunity and not let the "buy-in" process create an artificial barrier to that opportunity. Additionally, s/he must keep in mind that regardless of what value is established for the practice at the start of the associateship process, when the point is reached at which the original practitioner is giving up 50% of the ownership, his/her remaining 50% will be more valuable than 100% ownership was at the beginning of the process.

The economic opportunities to be captured through mergers are similar to those produced by successful associateships, but in the merger process, the timeline for capturing opportunity is much shorter because the patient volume necessary for achieving the desired end results is already in place. A financial opportunity equal to the fifth year associateship results shown in *Table 8.3* of our example would typically be achievable in the first year of a merger. If two practices exactly like the one in our example were to merge, the doctors would have the potential opportunity of increasing their salaries by 72.34% virtually "overnight" — from $137,215, to $236,483. Even if, in the process, they were to increase the number of key staff and, thus, increase fixed costs, a merger amongst two or more solo practices should result in a substantial improvement in profit for each practitioner by the end of the first year – especially given the power of today's technology to facilitate efficiency.

One would think that mergers would be frequent occurrences, especially given the extent of the opportunities to be captured and the number of one and two doctor practices still in existence. Constraints to forming mergers seem to be less related to business and technological challenges than to "human issues" — factors such as inertia, incompatible practice styles, previous personality clashes, unequal productivity, or fear of such things as losing control or autonomy. Even when potential business opportunities are compelling, the process is often derailed as a result of relatively small disagreements over practice valuation or compensation formulas. It is amazing to see doctors unable to agree over a few thousand dollars when millions are at stake – when a merger could increase profit margins substantially for all doctors, relative to the size of their disagreements!

In addition to the economic issues discussed here, I expect that future healthcare reform initiatives will create even more compelling clinical and financial reasons for adding associates and/or merging practices. Fortunately, there are already enough good economic reasons for initiating this process today. Those who have an understanding of the "profit margin opportunity" should be able to quantify the gains available to them and determine whether a particular opportunity makes sense for their practices.

Lessons in Efficiency from Nature

Much has been written about the advantages and disadvantages of group practice. If the changes in healthcare delivery currently predicted by experts come to fruition, the advantages of group practice will increase and "bigger will be better." Optimum group size has always been a topic of debate – generating a wide range of opinions based on subjective as well as objective data. As this debate continues, I feel that biology, as it relates to organisms found in nature, can offer us some interesting insight into the value of "size" as it might apply to medical groups.

I find it interesting that as an organism in nature increases in size, it requires less energy, per gram of tissue, to function properly. This tendency continues as we scale up in size from single celled organisms to the largest whales. As an example, let us compare an elephant's metabolism to that of a mouse. The elephant is 100,000 times bigger, yet its basal metabolic rate is only 7,000 times greater. Stated differently, the metabolism of one gram of mouse tissue is approximately fourteen times greater than that of one gram of elephant tissue. This is but one demonstration of the fact that the larger the organism, the more efficiently it functions at the cellular level. If this were not the case, the elephant's metabolism would be fourteen times greater than it is, and as a result, its life span would be much shorter. Just imagine what would occur if all organisms were as equally inefficient at metabolizing as mice! For one thing, food resources would be quickly depleted – in much the same way that financial resources are being depleted in order to support today's inefficient healthcare delivery system.

For the past fifteen years, as I worked to improve efficiencies in group practices, one consistency I observed is that efficiency improves only when science and mathematics (such as physics and statistics) are applied throughout the practice building process. The majority of processes utilized in a medical practice are dependent on efficient workflow (workflow of patients, information, and paper), and these "flows" all obey the laws of physics and mathematics. Technology has expanded the potential to apply these laws optimally because it enables work to be done where it makes the most sense, creating the opportunity to streamline and seamlessly connect process tasks, regardless of whether a portion of the work is being done in a treatment room, at a nursing station, in the billing office, at check-in or check-out counters, or even at locations physically removed from the office.

Much new information regarding "efficiency in nature" is being compiled in the fields of fractal geometry and fractal mathematics – both derived from Chaos Theory. The "rules" being revealed can be used to effectively reengineer medical practices. While I know of no comparable elephant/mouse examples in medicine – say, a group practice functioning at fourteen times the efficiency of a single doctor practice – the fact that such a model exists in nature presents the possibility that a comparable model might be developed in arenas such as ours.

Some medical groups are vastly more efficient than others. The individual doctors in practices that have been merged, completely ignoring the laws of physics, end up worse off than when they practiced solo; they capture none of the efficiencies that can be attained from coming together. Going back to our example in nature, we see a consistent relationship between "size" and "efficiency;" both animals and plants uniformly follow the "scaling laws" exhibited in nature. Living organisms routinely utilize the most efficient processes available to deliver resources, such as food and oxygen, to wherever they are needed at the cellular level. I think that we go wrong in the business world by not doing the same. Instead, we attempt to "build elephants using mouse tissue." An example of this is a group of doctors who in merging their practices attempt to retain all the attributes of their previous individual practices. The results of this strategy are not efficient – no more than they would be for organisms in nature, because this captures only one of the advantages of size – visibility. This type of grouping is occasionally found in nature and is used primarily as a protective mechanism. An example is when hundreds of sardines swim together in a tightly packed formation, giving the illusion that they are one large fish. Obviously, the metabolism of this "large fish" is great, being the sum total of the metabolism of the thousands of individual fish of which it is composed. One can easily see the difference between the efficiency of this large school of fish and one orca of "equivalent size." Compared to the group of sardines, the orca has the efficiency advantages of a large organism along with its intimidating size and structure, both of which serve it well in the environment in which it must compete.

If you are contemplating the creation or growth of a group practice, it is critical that you recognize from the beginning that "grouping" must be done with efficiency and scaling "laws" in mind. Recognize that you actually want to create a different and larger animal – not simply connect a group of similar small animals, forming the illusion of a large group. Doing so, you would only end up with "an elephant built using inefficient mouse tissue;" your result would be "a decrease in life quality and a shortened lifespan."

Know too that a group of twenty-five doctors is no more the same species as a group of four doctors than it is the same as a single doctor practice, and its support infrastructure is vastly different. The proverbial $64,000 question is whether it is possible to achieve the ten to fifteen fold efficiency advantages in medical groups that can be obtained in nature when optimum size is reached. My guess is that this would take an unbelievable level of commitment from the doctors in the group, strict adherence to the principles of physics and mathematics, knowledge of scaling laws, and a significantly large size. Even if a multiple of ten or fifteen represents the "impossible goal," a mere two or threefold improvement in efficiency would fix the high cost problems that plague most practices today. If your new "efficient animal" is designed with the attributes of an orca in mind, rather than a group of sardines, your group will have what it takes to become a more aggressive player in both today's and tomorrow's competitive healthcare environments.

Avoid Group Decision Pitfalls

It is often difficult for large groups to run efficiently and profitably because of the approach they take when making financial decisions. When considering the addition of any new expense to practice overhead, a sound business practice is to first conduct a cost-benefit analysis of that expenditure. This analysis will not be as straight forward for a group as it is for a solo practitioner or for doctors in a small group. The larger the group, the more important it is to question and ask before spending, "Who pays for this expenditure, and who benefits?" When the group is paying, but only a few members of the group will benefit, irrational behaviors can unintentionally creep into the decision-making process – behaviors that ultimately result in excessively high overheads. Simply being aware that this can happen and how it happens will help a practice capture far more of its potential efficiencies and avoid excessive costs. To aid your group in avoiding missteps when making financial decisions, let us take a look at several typical scenarios in which groups make suboptimal financial decisions.

Determining what is best for the individuals in a group versus what is best for the group as a whole is a potential source of contention when a group is making a decision. A common decision facing a medical group is whether to cover costs for a member doctor who wants to travel to a seminar for necessary CME credits – an amount that can vary widely. For example, let us assume that a doctor has projected fees of $4,000 for attending a "ski" seminar – including air travel, hotel accommodations, auto rental, seminar tuition, restaurant dining, and entertainment. Some might consider this exorbitant, and this is a substantial amount – far more than this doctor might have considered spending were he a solo practitioner. If the group is paying, and the group is large, the expense is often authorized because it requires a relatively small contribution from each member. The problem is that these "small" amounts accumulate over time, eventually adding up to large costs because every doctor member will expect a similar "perk" at some time in the future.

Another challenge is keeping the individual egos of the doctors in check when they are making decisions for the group. For example,

I recall working with an eight-doctor practice in which each doctor had a spacious, "Taj Mahal," private office. Because one doctor in the group had initially been adamant about this "necessity," the others had capitulated and then, when egos became involved, followed suit. Coming in as a consultant, I found that the group's greatest constraint to achieving greater productivity was a shortage of treatment and casting rooms necessary for seeing patients efficiently and effectively. To alleviate this problem, the doctors were considering their typical strategy – a move to larger quarters – but fortunately, upon analysis, they determined that the substantial costs of construction and increased rent would be too high. They, therefore, decided to seek an alternative solution. A relatively simple observation, pointed out to them by an "outsider," demonstrated that the combined square footage of their private offices offered more than enough space for the clinical rooms they needed for growth and presented an obvious solution to their less than ideal productivity. Fortunately, in this instance, the doctors chose to put their egos aside and share private offices. This gave them the additional space they needed for clinical work, and the move increased the practice's productivity without increasing costs. These doctors had ultimately recognized what was best for the practice as a whole.

Another pitfall to be avoided when making decisions for a group is the effect of "out of sight, out of mind." In a large medical group, throughout the course of a normal working day, most business transactions are performed "elsewhere" – at a location out of the doctors' sight. When backlogs occur in tasks such as billing, appointment scheduling, or check-in/check-out, the tendency is to quickly hire an additional employee whose responsibility it is to reduce this backup. Again, because the cost of adding one more employee is relatively small when it is shared amongst the members of a large group, the incremental addition of personnel seems to have little financial impact on individual group members and, hence, becomes the "easy fix" for backlogs.

Too often, no one in the group actually monitors these processes, and this belief that work is falling behind because of a shortage of personnel is usually erroneous. Rather, the situation is generally a result of process inefficiencies (which include unnecessary tasks, extended waiting time between linked tasks, and avoidable errors which must be identified and fixed at a later date). It is far easier for the group to simply apply more staff to backlogs than it is for them to thoroughly analyze their processes to find the source of backlogs and, upon discovering them, undergo the disruption required to make process changes that will fix them.

Due to the cumulative effect of multiple inefficiencies and the lack of effective decision making in dealing with them in some practices, wide variations develop in staffing ratios amongst groups having the same patient volume and/or similar gross revenues. I have seen some group practices with ratios as lean as two to three FTEs per doctor that function more effectively than ones with ratios as high as ten. As a matter of fact, a practice with a ratio of ten is typically far less efficient than one with three, and paradoxically, the often-heard lament of employees in these overstaffed groups is that they are "understaffed and need more help." Doctors seldom recognize this inverse relationship between staffing ratios and efficiencies. When the members of a group do not identify and deal with the inefficiencies that actually cause backups in their practice, the result is an excessively large expense in salaries – with marginal benefit. Because virtually all business operations in a large practice are out of sight, this problem is magnified in the business office, and an effective decision making process becomes critical to maintaining optimum processes at reasonable cost.

Even when there is no formal process in place, doctors making individual decisions typically weigh the cost and benefit of expenditures before making them. The value of performing a cost-benefit analysis when making practice expenditure decisions is obvious. Remember that what is not so obvious (and doctors need to keep this in mind) is that, in a group practice, this analysis can become skewed because it is individuals who are making the group's decisions, and what might make financial sense for any one individual may not be best for the group as a whole.

Practicing in a Group Can Increase Success and Happiness

The terms "happiness" and "success" are intimately connected – often mentioned in the same sentence. Conducting an Internet search shows us that this connection occurs hundreds of thousands of times. There is a profusion of book titles with this recurrent theme, books such as: *Achieving More Happiness and Success*, *Templeton's 21 Steps to Happiness and Success*, *Buy Keys to Happiness and Success*, and *The Secrets of Happiness and Success*. Happiness and success mean different things to each of us, and there is a wide range of what we each consider "happy" or "successful" to be. Authors write entire books attempting to grasp just what these words mean, but it is often easier for us to define them by their absence. There is definitely a connection between success and happiness, but cause and effect can be argued; does happiness lead to success – or does success lead to happiness? Depending on which you believe to be true, your approach to practice success (whatever that may be) could be enhanced.

According to psychology professor Sonja Lyubomirsky, a researcher of "happiness" at UC Riverside, "Happy people are more productive and make more money. They have more friends, and their marriages last longer. They're healthier and more creative, helpful, generous, and disciplined." While this seems like common sense, it doesn't get to the matter of cause and effect. One particular study cited by Professor Lyubomirsky captured my attention. This study was conducted using a group of people, half of whom watched a funny movie and half of whom did not, before being given a problem to solve. 75% of the subjects who had first watched the funny movie were able to solve the problem, as compared to only 13% of those who had not. Even if the results of this study were off by a wide margin, they would still be significant enough to interest anyone who wants to enhance his/her problem solving skills.

Success in today's rapidly changing medical environment requires that doctors overcome obstacles along the way, and this, in turn, requires the ability to solve problems. The above study certainly indicates that you will be more likely to find solutions to problems if you are "happy," which is decreasingly likely in today's healthcare environment in which internal and external factors are combining to make doctors less than happy with the practice of medicine. Because Professor Lyubomirsky's study suggests that happiness may be a factor leading to success in problem solving and because we need to solve problems on a daily basis in our practices, in addition to identifying the "hard" factors necessary for building a successful practice, we should also attempt to identify the "soft" factors that make us happy.

While there is a wide range in individual definitions of success and happiness, there are some universal consistencies that emerge which may help us in their pursuit. Certainly, money is included in most people's definition of success. Again, the range of what each of us considers "financial success" is wide, but each of us is likely to have a bottom line figure below which we would feel less than successful. Financial success certainly has some correlation with happiness, but is it happiness that leads to financial success, or is it "more money" that leads to happiness? Research does confirm the obvious – people living in wealthy nations are happier than those living in poverty stricken ones. But according to Ed Diener, a psychology professor at the University of Illinois who is a pioneer in happiness research and co-edited *Well-Being*, "All it takes is $8,000 a year, per capita, for money to stop being a factor in happiness." The 2000 Census showed the top median household income in the United States to be $56,300 (for those between the ages of 45 and 54). The lowest median income was $31,368 (for those between 65 and 74), and $41,414 (for the 25 to 34 year olds). I am sure that we all know many unhappy doctors earning substantially above all of these numbers. According to Diener, "Materialism is toxic for happiness." His studies indicate that even rich materialists aren't as happy as less well-off individuals who are not as concerned about "getting and spending."

Martin E.P. Seligman, a University of Pennsylvania psychologist and author of *Authentic Happiness*, has stated in *USA Today* that, "The happiest people spend the least time alone. They judge themselves by their own yardsticks, never against what others do or have." This shouldn't surprise anyone. We all grew up being taught that "keeping up with the Joneses" was not the road to happiness; yet, many doctors seem to adhere to this path of "keeping up." Research shows that people are not very good at predicting what will make them happy. Many pursue things they think will make them happy, but happiness becomes elusive. In spite of a wide range of opinions amongst individuals regarding what happiness and success are, there are recurring consistencies and correlations upon which most "happiness experts" agree, correlations of which we should be aware because they are relevant to our practices.

According to combined research, the happiest people have good friends, are engaged in absorbing activities, and are doing what they do best. This sounds a lot like the ingredients for a successful medical group practice to me. The activities in a group practice are just as absorbing as they are in solo practice, but being a member of a group allows each doctor to experience friendship in the workplace and to focus on his/her individual treatment preferences, skills, and strengths – on areas in which s/he is most interested and capable. Because there is a strong correlation between what we are good at and what we like to do, this presents a win-win that is good for our patients as well as ourselves. There are a number of sound business reasons why group practices make sense, but this aspect of happiness adds a whole new dimension.

Chapter 9

Eliminate Psychological Barriers to Practice Improvement

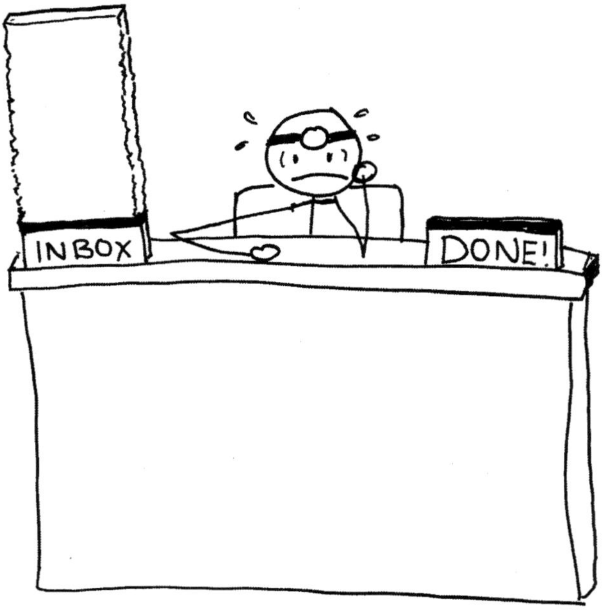

Don't Procrastinate

Procrastination is one of the prime causes of inefficiency and poor quality in a business. Samuel Clemens once said that the secret to success is getting started, but isn't there always a good excuse for putting things off? If Clemens is correct, following our "natural" tendency to procrastinate will negatively impact our level of success. This is especially true in today's changing healthcare environment, one that requires rapid response to frequent change.

As students, most of us have had the experience of putting off assignments until the last minute, at which time we rushed to get them done. If we ended up turning in an assignment late, or if we didn't have the time to give it our best effort, we suffered the consequence of a lower grade. In spite of having endured such negative experiences, many of us still tend to procrastinate. Today, we are running busy practices and depend on associates, advisors, and support staff to help us get work done. Unlike school, our success in practice is not only impacted by our own tendency to procrastinate, but also by this tendency in those working along side us. The year I was president of a professional association, I was stunned when I attended meetings and found that board members had sometimes not even begun assignments that they had agreed to have complete by the meeting dates.

Better management of our human instinct to procrastinate can make a dramatic difference in the economics and quality of a practice. A study conducted by Dan Ariely, of MIT's Sloan School of Management and Klaus Wertenbroch, of Insead in Fontainebleau, France, can help us understand how we can achieve this end. These researchers found that procrastination has much to do with how we set deadlines. They conducted a series of experiments in which participants were given a complex proofreading assignment. The first group was given a deadline of three weeks to complete the project, the second was given a series of interim deadlines for completing portions of the project, and the third group was allowed to set a series of interim deadlines for itself. Participants were told they would receive ten cents for each error they found and would be penalized one dollar for each day of missed deadlines.

The results revealed dramatic differences amongst the groups in both completion time and quality of work. The first group (given a single deadline) performed the worst in both areas. Their work, on average, was completed twelve days late, and each found only 70 errors. The second group (given a series of interim deadlines) performed the best. Their work, on average, was 0.5 days late, and each detected 136 errors. The third group (setting its own interim deadlines) was in the middle. They averaged 6.5 late days and found 104 errors. Profit was not mentioned in the study, but I did the math to compare outcomes. Members of Group One lost $5.00 (earning $7.00 in revenue for finding 70 errors and losing $12.00 in "fines" for being 12 days late), each member of Group Two achieved $12.60 in profit (earning $13.60 in revenue and losing $1.00 in fines), and those in Group Three produced $3.90 in profit (earning $10.40 in revenue and losing $6.50 in fines). In business terms, group one is out of business, while group two outperformed group three by 67%.

Judging from my experience, I see strong parallels between the findings of this study and the real world. There are thousands of medical practices outperforming the average profit level by 67%. Many are doing much better. One consistency I see in practices that achieve high profit levels is that their doctors make fast decisions, which they implement with minimal procrastination. It is clear from the above study that setting interim deadlines for your staff and associates will be a far superior approach to a single deadline or self determined, interim deadlines. The next time you find yourself setting a single deadline, such as, "I need this completed in two weeks," re-think your strategy. There are too many important goals that need to be met quickly, with no room for procrastination.

It's Okay to Start Small

Most of us would agree that the difficult part of any project is getting started. This is certainly the case for doctors who are struggling to improve practice profitability in the face of lower fees, higher costs, and greater patient volumes. An attempt to achieve a substantial increase in profit can seem so overwhelming that most practitioners end up doing nothing at all. One way to overcome this inertia is to focus on a number of "smaller" goals rather than one large, seemingly insurmountable one. This approach is less daunting and can yield significant results. For example, improving a practice's net profit by one third might appear to be "mission impossible"; however, if we, instead, set our goal as improving the performance of three of our processes by only 5% each, the task may now seem "doable." Let us take a closer look at one such "manageable" scenario.

Assume a typical solo practice with the following one year's financial statistics: 1) gross charges of $700,000, 2) a collection ratio of 40.6% – resulting in collections of $284,200, and 3) expenses of $170,236. Assume also that this doctor's goal is to improve profit by 33% – a task that feels overwhelming. What if, instead, s/he were to set a goal of improving the performance of several processes by only 5% – ones that impact charges, collections, and expenses? Might this be a more achievable goal? A 5% improvement in the three areas listed in *Table 9.1* would achieve the original "big" goal – a 33% increase in profit – from $113,964 to $151,606.

Table 9.1: Profit Increase Achieved by a 5% Improvement in Three Processes

	Before	% Change	After
Charges - a	$700,000	5%	$735,000
Collection Ratio - b	40.6%	5%	42.6%
Collections (a)(b)	$284,200	10%	$313,331
Expenses - c	$170,236	(5%)	$161,724
Profit (a)(b) – c	$113,964	33%	$151,606

Achieving this level of change requires three things: 1) the desire to make changes, 2) the establishment of achievable improvement targets, and 3) a commitment to see the project through to the end. Attaining a thirty three percent profit improvement (as in the above example) is not as difficult as it might seem. For example, to increase the total charges (the first 5% change in our table), the doctor and staff could focus on capturing all the charges for work already being performed by the practice. Most physicians "lose" over five percent of their total charges simply by: 1) not marking all billable services, 2) under-coding, and/or 3) "losing" charges – some superbills simply "fall through the cracks." In addition to increasing total charges, correcting these errors will also impact the collection ratio (our table's second 5% change). Increasing this ratio by five percent is not a difficult target to hit, especially when an electronic medical record or electronic superbill is implemented (on average, this alone increases a practice's collection ratio by seven percent).

The third savings in *Table 9.1* – decreasing expenses by five percent – is the most difficult of our example's three goals to achieve; however, most companies consider a cost reduction of ten percent easily doable – without hurting quality. A good place to begin when determining how to decrease costs is to consider the fact that the highest costs in a medical practice are staff salaries. This valuable resource (staff) should be used effectively; yet, it has been estimated that, on average, 16% of an "average" staff's time is spent dealing with paper (locating, distributing, and filing it). For this reason, it is easy to attain a five percent reduction in wasted staff time through implementation of information technology alone. Recognition of this fact and altering processes so that the entire staff is utilized more effectively will result in reduced costs and/or increased productivity.

While I have limited this example to strategies aimed at improving the performance of three processes by only 5%, many more strategies applicable to additional processes are available to us. Know that while a 5% improvement in just these three processes is an achievable goal, hitting a 7.5% improvement in these same three processes would not be significantly more difficult, and the outcome of a 7.5% process improvement would result in a whopping 50% increase in profit (see *Table 9.2*).

In this example, a 7.5% improvement in all three areas results in a practice profit increase of $56,997! Approaching our goals in this way – breaking them down into smaller, more manageable steps – gives us the courage to undertake change, a process that can yield "big" results. Streamlining processes and reducing errors are both within the reach of any practitioner who seeks improvement, and instituting a number of small process changes ultimately gives us the big end results we are striving for.

Table 9.2: Profit Increase Achieved by a 7.5% Improvement in Three Processes

	Before	% Change	After
Charges - a	$700,000	7.5%	$752,500
Collection Ratio - b	40.6%	7.5%	43.6%
Collections (a)(b)	$284,200	15.6%	$328,429
Expenses - c	$170,236	(7.5%)	$157,468
Profit (a)(b) - c	$113,964	50.0%	$170,961

For sports enthusiasts, a comparable situation can be found in baseball – one that helps to demonstrate this concept. Consider the difference between two players, one with a batting average of .200 and another one with a .300. The difference may appear "small," because the "only" difference between the two is that the .300 batter achieves one more base hit every ten times at bat. In reality, the situation is that the .200 batter is on the verge of being cut from the team while the .300 batter is negotiating with management for an increase in salary. Although he is achieving just one more hit every ten times at bat, the .300 batter is 50% more successful at getting on base than the .200 hitter. In baseball, as in business, "just a little more" can sometimes be substantial.

Use Retreats to Plan Big Changes

One truism that I have found throughout my career is that there is not always a correlation between the amount of work required to reach a goal and the size of the achievement. It seems intuitive that spending more time and exerting a greater effort when planning changes would assure bigger and better results; yet, some of our most significant achievements are accomplished in less time and with less effort than smaller ones. This is not to say that changes happen automatically; to achieve significant goals, we must have a well thought out master plan. It is a shame that we often miss big opportunities and accomplishments because we are bogged down in the day-to-day small things, the struggles of "getting through" the typical busy day. Obviously, we have to deal with the day-to-day "busyness" of our practices, but we should make sure that we also take time to tackle the big goals.

I think most of us recognize that there is a significant difference between being busy and being productive. I remember watching a basketball game in which one of the announcers kept pointing to the effort that one player was putting forth. Even though this player had not scored a point, or retrieved a rebound, he did appear to be putting out a major effort. Bill Walton, the co-announcer, was less impressed with this player's effort, remarking, "Don't confuse effort with accomplishment."

A business example that parallels this is that of the sales person who complains to his boss that he is underpaid, supporting his request for a raise with the explanation that he puts in more time and effort than his colleague in the adjacent cubicle who is much higher paid. He shows his boss phone logs, pointing out how he has made more than one hundred calls, while the higher paid salesperson has made only three. The statistic relevant to the boss, however, is that the "underpaid" salesperson has made one sale whereas the "overpaid" one has made three. In this case, the "underpaid" employee is confusing effort with accomplishment. This argument of "I am working harder and, therefore, should be paid more" is heard frequently in every business and is usually accompanied by numerous excuses for poor outcomes rather than attempts to discover why actual accomplishments have been few.

The primary reason that we miss opportunities or don't accomplish as much as we could is that we seldom have a "plan" for reaching our goals. Days pass quickly in a busy practice, and most decisions are directed at "putting out fires" and "getting through the day." Frequently, much of our work is even incomplete at the end of the day, necessitating that we catch up at a later time. It is impossible to set long-term goals and develop the strategy for achieving them in this type of environment. One solution to this dilemma is to get out of the routine office environment and devote a few days to contemplating "the big issues."

Many businesses set aside one weekend a year for a strategic planning retreat. Few medical practitioners, however, take this type of "time out." In spite of concerns regarding the added cost of a retreat, or the fact that you will be "giving up a weekend," this is a strategy worth adopting. A retreat is not the same as an office meeting, even when the meeting is off site. A retreat requires advance planning, and its significance is elevated when it is established as a priority, without overly skimping on cost. Sometimes it makes sense for attendance to be "doctors only", with the intent of setting this time aside for the purpose of establishing goals and priorities. At other times (such as prior to implementing a project which will require major change and full commitment from both doctors and staff), attendance should include the entire staff, along with the doctors.

The retreat environment is conducive to generating ideas, setting goals, and solidifying relationships amongst those who will ultimately be charged with prioritizing and implementing the plan that will be developed. Participants can relax, take time to envision the type of practice they would like to have, and set a plan for achieving this goal. It is best to set the bar high because this forces people to think out of the box and actually achieve "bigger" accomplishments. For example, if your goal were to grow profit by 10%, there would be a number of "easy" ways to achieve this; however, if the goal were to increase profit by 100%, you would have to be more creative, and this is best done in an atmosphere where no one is distracted by daily routine and everyone is encouraged to "think outside the box" – with no initial ideas being considered too radical. Once goals have been discussed and established at the retreat, a successful implementation is more likely upon return to the practice. This is because team members who have come together at the retreat have already "bought into" the plan; they have been instrumental in setting the goals and will be the ones charged with their implementation.

The first formal retreat held by the partners of my former practice was established with the purpose of setting goals for a major "re-computerization" of our office being contemplated for later in the year. The location we chose was a beach resort in California. In spite of the fact that the retreat included time for relaxing on the beach and social dinners in the evening, we emerged at the end of the weekend with clear written goals for our project and a formal plan of implementation. Instead of simply setting the typical goals for computerization (such as "becoming paperless"), we were able to set a number of broader ones designed to achieve specific results – including employment of this new system for improving quality (both service quality and quality of care) and increasing profitability (through both cost reduction and improved collections). If we had not held the retreat, we would have spent the same amount of money on technology and expended the same amount of time and energy installing and implementing it, but we simply would have achieved a "paperless practice" – with no improvement in either quality or profit.

One recommendation I make is that you "think big" during a strategic planning retreat; this is the time to be outrageous and think the impossible – the key to achieving big accomplishments. One thing that helps prepare participants for a retreat is reading motivational books prior to the event. These will not give you a specific plan, but they will help to "adjust" doctor and staff attitudes prior to the retreat so that the plan that is ultimately adopted will deliver bigger results. A book that I recommend is *The Magic of Thinking Big*, one that I had forgotten about until I came across it recently while "reorganizing" my office. My copy was quite worn, but as I thumbed through its pages, I realized this was the one "positive thinking" book that I had chosen to keep because it had helped me to overcome the tendency to focus on all the reasons why something might not work or to look for excuses as to why something had not worked. This book was copyrighted in 1959; the version I owned was reprinted in 1973, and the price had I paid for it was $1.50! I am sure it has gone through a number of revisions since then, but you or your staff should find this (or a similar book) an inspiring read prior to a retreat.

At your next office meeting, suggest the idea of scheduling a retreat for the purpose of addressing the long-term goals of your practice. Make this a high priority; pick a date when most everyone can attend; seek ideas for a location, and make it an event that everyone will look forward to. During the months leading up to the event, everyone will begin to think of ideas or issues s/he would like to discuss at the retreat. It is O.K. to list these and have a structured agenda, but leave a majority of the time open for "brainstorming sessions" at which everyone has a blank page in front of him/her with no preconceived point of view. If time is regularly set aside for this type of activity, you will find that your practice's accomplishments will be "bigger and better" each year.

Separate the Vital Few from the Trivial Many

Following office meetings, or successful retreats, multiple ideas are put forth, creating a long list that needs to be reduced to a manageable size. The challenge lies in deciding where to focus first. When facing this type of decision, it is helpful to be familiar with the "80:20 business rule," a concept that was initially derived by Vilfredo Pareto, an Italian economist born in 1906, who described the unequal distribution of wealth in his country in which 20% of the population was shown to hold 80% of the wealth. This finding was applied to business in the 1930s, when Joseph Juran, one of the early gurus focused on quality, determined that 20% of the defects in manufacturing caused 80% of its problems. As has been verified by multiple researchers, this 80:20 relationship is universal and holds true for most types of business decisions we face.

Examples of this 80:20 rule found in a medical practice include the likelihood that: 1) 20% of your staff cause 80% of your problems, 2) 20% of your staff provide 80% of your production, 3) 80% of your revenue is generated during 20% of your office hours, 4) 80% of your revenue comes from 20% of your patient visits, 5) 80% of your revenue comes from 20% of your CPT codes, and 6) 80% of your costs are generated by 20% of your expense categories. A slight variation on this theme is detected when implementing a large project. In most cases, a combination of the first 10% and last 10% of a project consume 80% of the project's total time. You may have experienced this if you have been involved in a home remodeling project. This is the reason that many construction companies run out of money when finishing the last 10% of a project.

Obviously, if you plan to focus on finding ways to increase productivity in your practice, you will first want to identify the 20% of patient visits, CPT codes, productive staff, and key hours that account for 80% of your revenue. This is certainly not an exhaustive list; there are many other factors impacting productivity that have been discussed throughout this book. The key point is that, in today's computerized medical practices, doctors face information overload. The amount of data generated by computers can be overwhelming, making it difficult to know where to focus attention. Understanding this Pareto concept and knowing that 80% of this data is basically "trivial" should give you confidence to narrow your focus to the 20% of "vital few" data that most significantly impact your practice.

Don't Become Discouraged when Starting a Large Practice Improvement Project

The graph that results from measuring and plotting the results of any new project's implementation in a medical practice will be a variation of an S curve. An understanding of this growth pattern will assist you in planning projects and managing them in a way that will help you to achieve maximum return on your investment.

The "S Curve"

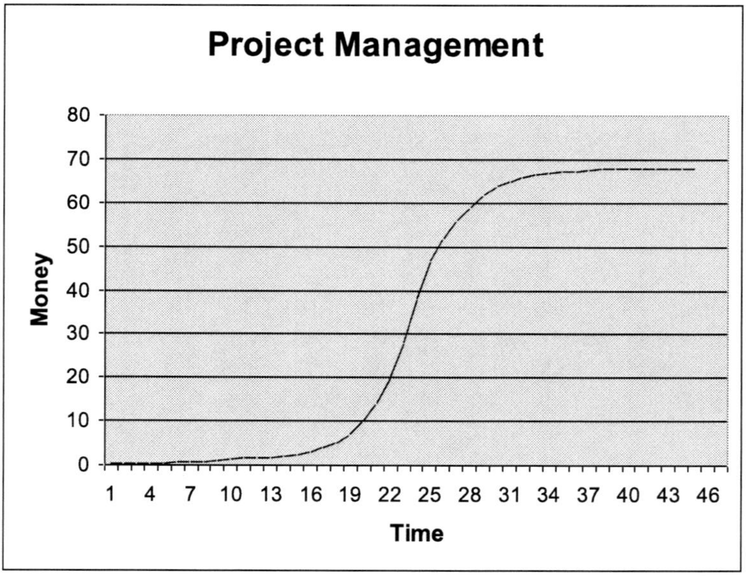

In the course of a business project, an S curve is produced when some quantity, such as cumulative cost, revenue, or volume of services, is plotted against time. The name is derived from the S-like shape of the curve, which is flat at the beginning and end and steep in the middle. The diagram above shows a typical S curve in which *Money* (the amount of reward) is plotted against *Time* (the period of time over which effort is expended). At the beginning, the curve is slow and deliberate, but in the "middle," it accelerates rapidly – eventually ending in deceleration as the project is completed and approaches the point at which the effect of "diminishing returns" sets in. The steepness of the slope and the eventual magnitude at its end point are, in large part, determined by how well the beginning, or "slow phase," is implemented.

Projects are most challenging at the onset, the time when money is going out and a significant amount of effort is being expended – with no evidence of positive return. If the project is a large one, this early phase can be long, disruptive, and frustrating – possibly even resulting in discontinuation of the project. Because this early phase is challenging, participants are tempted to "short circuit" or "cut corners" in an attempt to accelerate the process; however, shortening this early phase prematurely can have a deleterious effect on the steepness of the slope in the "middle" portion of the curve (where effort is the most productive) and on the ultimate height of the curve (which represents the total financial return on the investment).

Mathematicians attribute the cause of the initial "flat" phase of this curve to "starting friction." The "price of entry" is measured as the length of the distance from the starting point to the point at which the curve starts to accelerate upwards. For most people, this "price" presents a formidable barrier to ever even starting a project. This is especially true for medical practice projects when the investment of "time" required in the early phase is the doctor's time. If the physician does not recognize the importance of expending sufficient time and effort during this phase, results will be sub-optimal or the project may, possibly, even end in failure.

The implementation of new technology – such as an electronic medical record – is an example of a difficult project for a medical practice. This project requires research, goal setting, selection of technology, timeline planning, investment in hardware and software, doctor and staff training, data conversion, and eventual implementation. There is no question that short circuiting the initial stages (investing too little time in research, planning, training, and physician involvement) will have a negative impact on the eventual height of the S curve. If the doctor(s) and staff are not committed to putting the necessary time and effort into the beginning phase, it is better that the project not be undertaken at all. If a doctor fails to understand the importance of this initial phase of a project, it will be difficult for him/her to tolerate the extended period of disruption during which effort and money are expended with little sign of return.

The extent of the eventual project "pay-off" is in direct proportion to the effort expended in preparing and building infrastructure throughout the early phase. The middle portion of the S curve represents the "productive" phase of a project. This is when the results of the effort expended during the early phase are realized. What helps a doctor make it through the difficult early phase is a strong belief that no matter how challenging the initial phase may be, s/he will eventually reach this middle phase, and the end results will be more than worth the effort. Much of this confidence is built throughout the early research and planning of the project, when the doctor takes the time to set goals and gain a thorough understanding of precisely how his/her project will result in the achievement of the goals s/he envisions.

This upward curve eventually flattens out. This is the point at which all major project goals have been achieved, and the return-on-effort diminishes. At this point, a program of continuous improvement – seeking small, incremental improvements over the long-term – should be instituted. Continuous improvement becomes part of everyday operations. This requires far less effort than the original project and causes little disruption. If a continuous improvement process is not put in place, there is a chance that complacency will follow, and the S curve might eventually go into decline.

It is important to recognize that any type of project creates change, and that even small changes can be difficult to deal with. It is also important to recognize that all projects go through some type of S curve throughout their "life cycles" – even relatively small ones, such as purchasing a new piece of equipment or implementing a new service. Superior project results are most likely to be achieved when the participants are aware of and understand this S curve phenomenon. With this understanding, it is more likely that the necessary amount of time and money will be expended during the early phase of change and that participants will "stick with" a project, regardless of the disruption and/or obstacles that are encountered along the way. Confidence in the belief that their projects will eventually be successful will help doctors and staff to see them through to the top of their S curves.

Track Your Improvement

For virtually every human endeavor – ranging from a simple game to complex business operations – participants seek benchmarks for setting standards whereby they can evaluate their performance. Each benchmark conveys a limited snapshot of important information and should be considered in conjunction with others to form a more complete picture. Similar to the fact that taking X-Ray views from different angles allows a more accurate interpretation of each individual film, the best overall interpretation of a medical practice's performance is gained through investigation of a combination of relevant benchmarks.

To be of practical use, benchmark values must accurately differentiate average from superior performance. Often, this is not the case. When I was a child, the benchmark for identifying optimum blood pressure was considered to be "one hundred plus your age." A fifty year old with a blood pressure of 145 was considered to be in excellent health. The problem with applying this benchmark value today is that it depicts the average American of a previous time who was likely to smoke, eat a high fat diet, and rarely exercise. A significant segment of our current population is non-smoking, eats less meat, and exercises regularly. The old benchmark "normal" values would be seen as pathologic for today's new "superior" group. Many medical practice management benchmarks currently being cited are similarly outdated and misleading. They represent practices that could now be considered inefficient and "out of shape." Old standards no longer apply to the current needs of medical practices; some long-standing benchmarks once thought to be "superior" may now actually represent "pathology."

The Medical Group Management Association (MGMA) and other organizations regularly publish medical office statistics and benchmarks, but much of this data is representative of average, inefficient medical practices. Over several decades, I have had the opportunity of working with practices throughout the country. Many of these are part of an emerging subset of healthier practices that are setting radically new standards. The good news is that these practices are achieving success through use of strategies that are readily available to all physicians. In spite of low fees and the concurrent increase in complexity in the practice of medicine, many of these doctors are ethically earning two to three times that of the average physician, and in spite of their lower cost structures, they are maintaining a high quality of patient care and satisfaction. While developing and implementing strategies for making their practices equivalent to this superior group of practices, doctors must have relevant benchmarks against which to measure and track their performance.

Medical practitioners and their staffs can achieve the greatest gains in performance by focusing on activities that result in efficiency and productivity improvement. To determine the effectiveness of their efforts, they must have benchmarks against which to measure both efficiency and productivity. I find the following six benchmarks to be a good starting point for assessing a practice and measuring performance: 1) profit increase relative to revenue increase, 2) the number of FTEs per doctor, 3) the collection ratio, 4) the cost per patient, 5) the revenue per patient, and 6) patient waiting time. These six benchmarks are easy to calculate using data readily available in most practices, and when considered together, they will provide a good assessment of how a practice is performing and where it can be improved.

Profit Increase Relative to Revenue Increase

Growth is a natural outcome for businesses that provide valuable products or services, and private medical practices are no exception. Doctors who are rendering quality care will develop good reputations with ever-increasing numbers of patients coming to their offices. A practice's revenue increases along with this growth; unfortunately, so do the expenses and the complexities of "doing business." The percentage of this revenue increase that ultimately translates into profit is dependent on the practice's level of efficiency; an efficient practice will capture a greater percentage of revenue growth as profit than an inefficient one. Doctors incorrectly blame lower fees when growth has a lesser impact on profit, but failure to convert an increase in revenue into a commensurate level of profit is the result of managing increasing volume and complexity with inefficient processes. The percent of increase in profit relative to the percent of increase in revenue is an easy statistic to calculate, and tracking this statistic will help doctors improve their performance.

A sure sign of inefficiency in a growing practice is when revenue is increasing at a higher rate than profit. An efficient practice will produce at least the same percentage increase in profit as revenue. The superior, efficient practice can achieve a percentage increase in profit that is actually greater than that in revenue. The first example I encountered demonstrating how significant this phenomenon could be was a practice that had generated a revenue increase of 24% over the period of one year. This is a spectacular achievement by any standard. Unfortunately, a concurrent 36% overhead increase and 3% collection ratio decrease had resulted in a profit increase of only 6%. While the doctor was happy that profit had increased 6%, he realized that the 24% revenue increase should have resulted in a substantially higher increase in profit.

The tables below represent three separate practices, each experiencing a 10% growth in both volume and revenue. They demonstrate that, depending on each practice's level of efficiency, the impact of growth on expenses varies significantly and that this, in turn, impacts profit. Comparisons of the rates of increase in revenue to the rates of increase in profit for these practices reveals a clear pattern. In this example, the superior practice's rate of growth in profit is more than four times that of the inefficient one.

Profit: Before and After Reengineering Processes

Table 9.2: Inefficient Practice

	Before	After	% Increase
Revenue	$300,000	$330,000	10.0%
Expenses	$165,000	$189,750	15.0%
Profit	$135,000	$140,250	3.9%

Table 9.3: Efficient Practice

	Before	After	% Increase
Revenue	$300,000	$330,000	10.0%
Expenses	$165,000	$181,500	10.0%
Profit	$135,000	$148,500	10.0%

Table 9.4: Superior Efficient Practice

	Before	After	% Increase
Revenue	$300,000	$330,000	10.0%
Expenses	$165,000	$173,250	5.0%
Profit	$135,000	$156,750	16.1%

Suffice it to say, practices with superior levels of efficiency will be well positioned to convert a greater percentage of their growth into profit. Warren Buffett, one of the world's most astute investors, stated this concept well: "Great businesses make lousy investments if management cannot convert sales into profit. Managers of high-cost operations tend to find ways to continually add to overhead, whereas managers of low-cost operations are always finding ways to cut expenses."

FTE to Doctor Ratio

The FTE (Full-Time-Equivalent) staff to doctor ratio of a practice tells us more about that practice than the total dollar amount of its staff salaries. Salaries vary greatly by region or physician choice, making comparisons amongst practices unreliable. I focus on the FTE ratio because payroll accounts for the highest percentage of office overhead in most medical practices. Ideally, a doctor needs to determine the optimum staffing ratio – one that will deliver the highest levels of productivity, treatment quality, and patient satisfaction at the lowest cost. Reducing the FTE staff to doctor ratio is desirable only when it does not lower physician productivity, quality of care, or patient satisfaction. The typical practice utilizes obsolete business processes, establishing an environment in which, at any given point in time, 30% of the staff are idle waiting for something and 25% are performing unnecessary tasks. For this reason, most FTE ratios are significantly high, with no corresponding benefit. The fact is that smaller FTE ratios can actually be consistent with higher levels of productivity, higher quality, and lower costs.

Table 9.5 shows findings from the *NAHC* (National Association of Healthcare Consultants) *2000 Statistical Report*. This report should be more reliable than many others because the numbers are reported by accountants rather than self-reported by doctors. It compares closely to practices that I have independently analyzed.

Table 9.5: FTE Staff to Physician Ratio

Specialty	FTE to Physician Ratio
Ophthalmology	5.19
OB/GYN	4.35
Dermatology	4.30
Otolaryngology	4.22
Hematology/Oncology	4.19
Family Practice	4.18
Orthopedic Surgery	4.12
Cardiology (Invasive)	4.04
Pediatrics	3.79
Gastroenterology	3.75
Internal Medicine	3.51
Urology	3.29
Podiatry	2.94
Neurology	2.70
Surgery (General)	2.50

Typically, larger practices have high FTE ratios. Up to a point, higher ratios translate to higher productivity and greater earnings for doctors. Remember that each of these averages represents a range. Even though orthopedic practices at the time of this report had an average FTE staff to doctor ratio of 4.12, I have seen this ratio as high as ten in several large orthopedic groups. It is likely that neither an extremely high nor an extremely low ratio is optimal; however, it is safe to assume that the efficient benchmark is at least 30% lower than the averages listed in this table. For large, busier practices with FTE ratios well above average, efficient FTE benchmarks may be 50% lower than their current numbers. Again, Warren Buffett stated it well: "There is a right size staff for any business operation. For every dollar of sales, there is an appropriate level of expense."

Collection Ratio

The collection ratio reflects the efficiency and effectiveness of the entire billing process – from initial "error free" data entry and obtainment of treatment authorizations to co-pay collection, submission of claims, follow-up, and final deposit of payment. Tracking a practice's internal collection ratio over time and separately tracking the collection ratio for each third party payer are valuable exercises – especially when volume is increasing. Increasing the collection ratio should be a high priority for every practice. Obviously, every doctor would like to achieve a 100% collection ratio, but this is unrealistic. Because each third party payer uses its own fee schedule and rules for adjudicating claims, doctors often submit fees that are higher than those of the third party, knowing at the time that much of this money cannot be collected and will have to be adjusted at a later time. This results in inflated account receivables and artificially low collection ratios.

Because each doctor has a different "retail" fee schedule, it is not possible to directly compare collection ratios amongst practices other than as "reality checks" to see how they align. We can, however, compare practices that are on a common database because we can "normalize the collection ratio" by superimposing the same fee schedule on all practices. While it is revealing to know how you are doing relative to other practices in your specialty, the goal is to improve your own collection ratio. To accomplish this, it is essential that you be able to track your own progress, explain fluctuations, and measure results as you implement changes directed at improving this process.

The 2000 NAHC national database shows that the average medical practice collection ratio is 70.2% (from a sample size of 3,032) and that of the average surgical practice is 59.4% (from a sample size of 2,196). The average weighted composite for all physician practices is approximately 67%; however, at the time of this report there were excellent, highly profitable practices that collected less than 50% and financially struggling practices that collected more than 80%. Today, many practices utilize a schedule with fees that are 2.5 times the Medicare rate. If this were the standard for all practices, the actual outcome of collecting 40% of the total charges would be equivalent to a 100% collection rate. One consistency I find is that the collection ratio for an inefficient billing process is typically at least eight percentage points below where it should be. Ideally, we should strive to collect 100% of what we are *allowed* to collect. A good starting point for achieving this is to use a practice's historic rate and set a benchmark that is at least eight percentage points higher than that rate.

One benchmark that correlates well with a practice's collection ratio is the length of time that its money remains in accounts receivable. Faster money collection always translates to a higher collection ratio. Collecting cash (co-pays, deductibles, non-covered services, and the patient's portion of the insurance) and entering billing data on the day of service, making fewer mistakes, submitting claims to third parties quickly, and following up immediately on under-payments all speed the collection process and translate to higher collection ratios.

Revenue and Expense per Patient

Most practices use standard financial statements to monitor total practice revenue and expenses. While these give an indication of productivity and efficiency, they become even more useful when considered relative to patient volume. This can be accomplished easily by dividing total revenue or expenses by total patient volume, expressing these amounts as revenue, or cost, per patient.

A patient volume increase is likely to increase total costs, but the relevant benchmark is whether the cost *per patient* is increasing or decreasing. The goal should be to decrease cost per patient. This can be done either by actually reducing total costs (i.e. through a reduction in FTE staff per doctor) or by *relatively* reducing costs (i.e. spreading a greater patient volume over the same number of FTEs). Future medical practices based on collaborative models will have significant opportunities to create per patient cost reductions.

Waiting Time

A factor in the operations of a medical practice that most directly correlates with higher quality treatment and patient satisfaction is a decrease in the time a patient waits. Richard J. Schonberger, author of *Building a Chain of Customers*, states, "If there was one single measure of quality, especially quality of service, waiting time (or lack of it) is probably it." Patients want faster access to practices, and they dislike waiting at the office once they arrive. They are even willing to pay more for short waits and quicker access as evidenced by the success of many "concierge" practices.

It is difficult to reduce waiting time, and when you are attempting to do so, you must be able to accurately measure and monitor it so that you can set achievement benchmarks. Today's software can be used as a tool for accurately measuring wait time, and this will assist you in setting benchmarks. This is accomplished by "tagging" patients at critical times – when they arrive, when they are moved to treatment rooms, and when they check out. This tracking data provides a total breakdown and "count" of the patient's waiting time and is, therefore, useful for pinpointing exactly where office processes are breaking down.

Measuring waiting time is key to understanding the interrelationships amongst benchmarks because virtually every patient satisfaction issue and most quality of care issues are related to waiting time. A practice that demonstrates shorter patient waits and has a low FTE staff to doctor ratio is clearly a superior practice. One with high FTE ratios and long patient waits is not translating its large number of FTEs into higher quality. If we now compare the revenue and costs, per patient, we get an even more complete picture. The superior practice (the one with fewer FTEs *and* shorter waits) will be creating more profit per patient. It may accomplish this by being more productive (higher revenue per patient), more efficient (lower costs per patient) or ideally, both (the extreme superior practice). Tracking these benchmarks and setting the bar high will put a practice on a course capable of delivering the best care most profitably.

Chapter 10

Know the Value of Your Practice

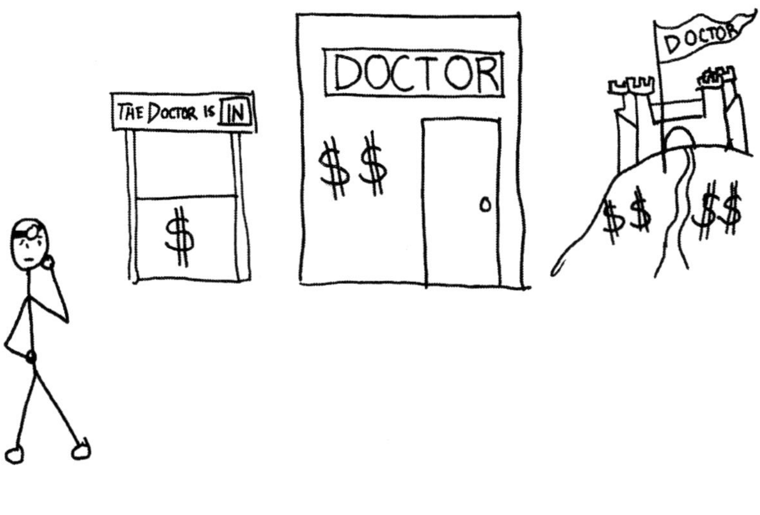

Practice Valuation Is Dependent on Both Buyers and Sellers

What is your practice worth? While value can be determined through a number of different methods and formulas, the reality is that no matter how "accurate" a valuation may be, price is ultimately negotiated. As when selling any type of business, regardless of the predetermined valuation, the selling price is ultimately what the buyer is willing to pay and the seller is willing to accept. Neither of these amounts necessarily correlates with "actual" value, but this is the reality of buying and selling a business.

The "open market sale" of a medical practice (when a solo practitioner is planning to retire and simply lists his/her practice for sale) presents a very different scenario from one in which the buyer is a current associate who, in anticipation of becoming a partner, is purchasing a percentage of the practice in which s/he is practicing or one where the associate is buying out the owner who wishes to retire. Many negotiations between associates and owners fall apart because the owner believes his/her practice is worth its weight in gold, while the associate takes the position that s/he should be given the practice outright. The problem usually boils down to the fact that neither party fully understands the other's point of view or, most importantly, the sources from which a practice's value are actually derived. It is imperative that negotiations be based on realistic evaluations. To buyers, valuation prices often appear to be "arbitrary" – resulting in hard feelings, breakdown of negotiations, and eventual dissolution of relationships that heretofore may have been amicable.

An interesting experiment conducted by Eric Johnson, co-director of the Center for Decision Sciences at Columbia University, gives valuable insight into why the perception of value can vary so widely between buyers and sellers. In this experiment, Johnson divided one of his classes into two groups, asking the first group how much they would pay for a coffee mug. The typical response he received was $4. He gave the second group the same mug for free and then asked, "How much would I have to pay you to part with it?" What is important to recognize at this point is that Johnson is basically asking the same question of both groups, which is, "How much is this mug worth to you?" Surprisingly, the average response from the second group was $8. Researchers refer to this phenomenon as the *endowment effect*, which Johnson explains in the following way: "Simply owning something increases its value."

This experiment can help us to understand why negotiations involving practice buy-in and buy-out situations are difficult and often defy logic. If two groups can disagree this much over the value of a simple coffee mug, it is no wonder that the difference in the perception between buyers and sellers of the value of a more complex entity such as a medical practice can be so extreme – with each party feeling that the other is being unreasonable. When negotiating price, it is helpful to understand that these issues of "behavioral economics" are an unspoken factor; yet, ultimately, practice valuation must be approached in an objective way, one that leads the buyer and seller to come to a reasonable agreement as to a practice's fair value.

Finding a Reasonable Middle Ground Between Buyer and Seller

Many doctors assume that practice value is determined solely by gross revenue. They may hear of a practice "selling" for a year's gross (or a percentage of a year's gross) and arbitrarily use this same measure for determining the buy-in or selling price for their own practices. Problems arise from the fact that the range of true value for practices with similar revenues can be extremely broad.

Consider two real examples. At one extreme, the owner of a practice grossing $700,000 was able to convince his associate to pay $350,000 for 50% of the practice. Problems inherent in this particular agreement were that the practice overhead (which had not been taken into account when negotiating) was $500,000, and the associate was not nearly as productive as the owner. Due to this combination of circumstances, the purchaser today does not earn enough from the practice to make a living, and legal action has ensued. At the other extreme, is a practice grossing $300,000. This practice was on the open market for over a year and never sold. A nearby practitioner offered $15,000 for the phone number alone, allowing the owner to sell the equipment separately. The result was that the purchaser's new patient volume increased by 400 patients a year – increasing his yearly net income significantly. The buyer was satisfied, and in spite of the fact that the seller received well below the practice's "actual value" (if determined by gross revenue), he too was happy just to get "something" for his practice and its equipment.

There are a myriad of ways to appraise a medical practice. My purpose here is not to teach all of these methods but to help the reader understand how various opportunities and risks can impact practice value, regardless of the appraisal method employed. It is helpful to have an understanding of the "Summation of Assets" approach to valuation. This approach is based on the philosophy that a practice has both tangible and intangible assets and that, if values for all identified assets can be agreed upon, the overall value of the practice can then be determined simply by totaling the value of all the assets.

Setting a price on tangible assets (such as clinical and business equipment, furniture, fixtures, instruments, supplies, leasehold improvements, the collectible portion of accounts receivable, and cash) is relatively easy and straightforward. These assets can be valued at book value, replacement cost, or fair market value, and as long as both parties agree on the method for determining price, evaluation of tangible assets can be objective and non contentious. What makes overall practice valuation difficult is appraisal of the intangible assets, and this is where the majority of a practice's value typically lies.

A practice's most significant intangible asset is "goodwill" which encompasses reputation, referral sources, medical records, and the cash flow that one expects to generate from these sources. "Goodwill" is an extremely valuable, difficult to acquire asset, and its evaluation is complex. Buyers and sellers will often be far apart in their perceptions of 1) what this asset is worth and 2) the opportunities and risks associated with retaining or even growing it. The extreme range of possible goodwill values accounts for the wide range of negotiated sale prices for practices that have the same, or similar, gross revenues.

Any valuation method used in a sale can be challenged. It is important to understand that even though value can be objectively determined through a variety of methods, sale price is ultimately negotiated and could vary substantially from appraised value. It is also essential to recognize that a wide range of outcomes may be satisfactory to both the buyer and the seller but that an acceptable outcome can only be derived if both parties understand the sources of the practice's value and the levels of opportunity and risk associated with each one. The ideal is to identify an overlapping area where the range of outcomes acceptable to both the buyer and seller intersect. The more clearly each party understands these sources of value and the better able each is to quantify the levels of opportunity and risk from the other's perspective, the less emotion will play a part in the negotiation process, and the better the eventual outcome will be for both.

Let us examine key factors that should be considered when determining price and identify potential opportunities and risks associated with each. The more aware both negotiators are of the factors impacting practice value, the easier it will be for each of them to come to an understanding of the other's perspective. This will also facilitate, when necessary, objective arguments as to what either the buyer or the seller sees as the opportunities and risks associated with the sale and whether these opportunities and risks are either larger, or smaller, than the other party perceives them to be.

Cash Flow

I stated earlier that a practice's gross revenue should not be the sole determinant of its value. Gathering financial information, including a number for gross revenue, should be the starting point for determining value because, when purchasing a business, what the buyer really is purchasing is a best guess of what that business's future cash flow will be. A factor that should be determined when setting price is the potential of future cash flow – is it expected to remain the same, increase, or decrease? Analysis should focus on 1) opportunities that provide the possibility of increased cash flow and 2) risks that might decrease cash flow.

It is good to begin a valuation by examining financial statements from the most recent three years. This will reveal historic trends in revenue, expenses, and profitability and will approximate the value of hard assets. From this historic base, valuation should then be focused on "finding" the sources of the practice's revenue and expenses. From here, analysis should focus on the opportunities and risks associated with the likelihood that, after the sale, each of these sources will continue on as before, increase, or decrease. While current profit is a significant statistic, a buyer needs to consider the potential for future profit. S/he may find that a practice presents possibilities for improved efficiency and, therefore, increased collections and reduced costs – resulting in higher future profit, even at the same patient volume – an opportunity. Another possibility: the buyer may discern that 1) overhead is extremely low, with a potential need for additional personnel, or 2) office rent is about to increase – either of which will reduce profit, thus making the practice less valuable to the buyer – a risk. All such possibilities must be addressed, and historic financial statements can help when assessing potential changes in outcomes.

A practice that generates "excess earnings" offers the most significant cash flow value to a potential buyer or incoming associate/partner. Excess earnings can be defined as the profit a practice achieves over and above the amount that a doctor entering into practice in a particular specialty can expect to earn. For example, if the average take-home for a doctor in a specific specialty is $220,000 a year, and the profit for a particular practice is $300,000, this practice could hire a doctor at $220,000 and have $80,000 left over as "excess earnings." This yearly $80,000 excess has a fair value that can be determined, and a doctor buying into this practice is acquiring this $80,000, per year, in addition to his/her $220,000 salary. One can calculate this value through a standard "present value" approach by projecting the cash flow into the future and discounting it back to present value using a discount rate that reflects the risk of the cash flow continuing. In many businesses, the cash flow would be projected out thirty or more years, but in medical practices, I typically project cash flow out five to seven years and discount it back using a 20% discount rate. Based on a standard present value formula, and projecting the excess $80,000 cash flow out five years, its present value would be $239,249.

Patient Base

The most significant assets a practice has to offer are its existing patient base and its new patient referral sources. Essential elements to consider when assessing the patient base are: 1) the total annual number of patient visits, 2) the annual number of new patients, and 3) the sources of new patients (i.e. physician referrals, patient referrals, community organizations, HMO contracts, PPO networks, public speaking opportunities, a website, advertising, and office signage). A few of the questions to consider when assessing volume include: 1) Are new patient referrals and patient volume increasing, decreasing, or remaining flat? 2) What is the probability that existing referral sources will continue, decline, or increase? 3) Are the HMO contracts transferable and the PPO networks open? and 4) Is the community growing? Regardless of whether you are the owner or the potential buyer, it is important to ask, or have answers to, questions regarding these issues, all of which can have a positive or negative impact on future patient volume. Together, these factors combine to create the complete picture of a practice. They provide objective information regarding potential risks and opportunities and the extent to which these risks and opportunities might be used to justify a given practice valuation.

One specific patient statistic that can be helpful to a buyer's analysis of practice volume is the new patient return ratio. This is found by dividing total patient visits, per year, by the number of new patients, per year. If a practice attracts 1,000 new patients and has 8,000 office visits yearly, the new patient return ratio is eight. The average ratio will vary by specialty, and it is an important number to know when determining the value of a practice. Because, in my particular specialty, the average ratio ranges between five and six, a practice with a ratio of eight presents fewer opportunities for future increases in volume (if new patient referrals remain the same) than a practice with a ratio of three or four. There is some risk to a buyer that this high ratio could decrease, depending on his/her practice style or ability to manage a higher than average patient load.

Payer and Employer Mix

Analysis of payer mix entails a breakdown of the percentages of all payers' contributions to total practice revenue (such as Medicare, Medicaid, Blue Cross, Blue Shield, HMOs, United Healthcare, HMOs, PPOs, and cash). Analysis of this mix should be limited to a practice's top ten payers. This will provide an idea of the degree to which the practice is dependent on specific individual payers. Analysis should also include the average collection ratio for each payer. This will allow comparison of the reimbursement rates of all third party payers for the purpose of determining the relative value of each to the practice.

It is also helpful for a potential buyer to obtain statistics regarding employer mix and attempt to correlate this information with statistics for payer mix. Information gathered should only include the largest employers. Results can be utilized for estimating risk (by finding companies whose growth rates are flat, or declining) and evaluating opportunities (by finding companies that are growing and/or are utilizing third party payers with reimbursement rates that are better than average). A doctor who wants to buy, or buy into, a practice and then increase patient volume can use this information as a guide for focusing his/her marketing efforts.

Revenue per Patient

Revenue per patient is a statistic critical to a potential buyer when s/he is evaluating opportunity and risk, and it can be calculated by dividing total yearly revenue by the total yearly number of patient visits. To understand why this number is important, assume you are considering the purchase of one of two practices in the same geographic area, each of which has annual collections of $500,000 and an overhead of $250,000. Both practices have received credible valuation reports, each supporting a price of $400,000. Assume that your calculation for the average revenue per patient for *Practice A* is $50.00 and that *Practice B's* is $150. This additional information indicates that these two practices are not of equal value.

Which practice delivers the greater opportunity upon purchase, and which one presents greater risk? Assume that average revenue, per patient, in this specialty is $100. Simply increasing *Practice A's* productivity to average would double its revenue, while increasing productivity above *Practice B's* current $150 per patient would be difficult. There is actually significant risk that this practice's productivity will drop, along with a strong possibility that the current practitioners are over-coding. Information derived from analysis of this critical statistic, can help a potential buyer determine these types of opportunities and risks which are inherent in the purchase of any practice.

Because revenue per patient is also strongly influenced by a practice's service mix, a potential buyer can enhance his/her analysis of risk and opportunity when considering purchase of a practice by listing specific services provided by that practice and then determining the percentage of the whole that each represents. For example, if a practice collects an average of $50 per patient, with the average in the specialty being $100, there may be specific services the doctor is not providing, or s/he may be under-coding. If so, this presents an opportunity for the new buyer to make the practice more valuable. If a practice, however, collects $150 per patient, there may be services or procedures the current doctor is providing which the new doctor may not be trained to perform, or does not wish to provide. If so, this would add risk and reduce the value of the practice to the buyer. A thorough way of evaluating a practice's overall service mix is to calculate both revenue per patient and the percentage that specific services represent of the whole.

Billing Practices

Analysis of the billing process is critical to practice evaluation as this process has a significant impact on both revenue and profit. A good way to begin examination of this process is to randomly sample charts and EOBs. It is important to determine whether the doctor is down-coding, up-coding, or coding correctly. Obviously, down-coding creates opportunity for future increases in revenue – supporting a higher value for the practice. Up-coding, on the other hand, adds risk and reduces a practice's value, because converting to correct coding would reduce revenue.

The number of CPT codes billed, per visit, is also an important statistic to examine when evaluating billing practices. This can be calculated by dividing the total number of procedures (found on the procedure report) by the total number of patient visits. If we assume that in a specific specialty, the average physician bills two CPT codes, per visit, a number below this represents opportunity, while a number above this represents potential risk.

There should be some correlation between the number of CPT codes billed, per visit, and revenue, per patient. For example, a doctor who bills an E/M code and an x-ray would require two CPT codes, and the revenue per visit should be higher than if only one service were provided. A doctor averaging 1.25 CPT codes per visit may be ignoring secondary patient complaints (which presents opportunity) while a doctor averaging 3.5 CPT codes per visit may be providing unnecessary services (presenting risk).

It is also helpful for a buyer to evaluate the efficiency and effectiveness of the billing process in order to determine room for potential improvement in the collection ratio (which increases profit). It is helpful in this determination to know: the collection ratio trends over the most recent three years, the average number of days receivables remain in A/R, the percentage of accounts that remain in A/R over 90 days, and the claim rejection rates. Thorough evaluation of these four factors should include close observation of the billing process, checking for efficiency. This should entail noting 1) whether co-pays and balances are collected at check-in (or check-out), 2) whether superbills are marked at the time of service, 3) the amount of time that passes before superbills are entered into the system, and (4) whether staff discusses fees with patients prior to initiating specific (especially costly) types of treatment. Significant delays and inefficiencies in the billing process represent opportunity for changes that would increase the collection ratio. This is something that will increase revenue without increasing patient volume.

Compensation Formulas

For the significant number of doctors who practice solo, determining their optimum compensation plan is a "non-issue." A solo practitioner's "formula" is basically that the amount of revenue left-over after all practice expenses are paid becomes his/her compensation; however, this basic "whatever is left" formula does not adequately address the contention that arises when two or more doctors practice together and disagree over how to fairly divide "leftover" revenue. Compensation concerns are encountered in several common situations – when independent doctors join together under one roof for the purpose of sharing resources and expenses (such as employees, space, equipment, and supplies), when associate doctors join existing practices as employees, when two or more doctors form a partnership, or when two or more practices merge.

A primary challenge to creating the optimum compensation formula is inherent in the fact that doctors are rarely "equals" in such things as their reputations, levels of productivity, patient volumes, payer mixes, office hours, investments in the practice, or practice management skills. A compensation formula must address all these differences – optimizing the needs of each individual involved, while at the same time meeting the goals of the group as a whole. There is no "one size fits all" formula that can deliver this outcome, and any one that is successful requires tradeoffs from everyone involved. The challenge in any negotiations regarding compensation is that each doctor will perceive the tradeoffs that s/he makes for the benefit of the group from his/her individual perspective. If any one doctor negotiates too good a "deal," creating winners and losers within the group, the formula, and perhaps even the group itself, will not last long. Even when all seem happy with their compensations, factors such as productivity, patient volume, and working hours will change over time and render a once well-working formula obsolete. Because of this reality, these formulas must be revisited and "tweaked" every few years to confirm that they still meet the needs of the group.

An ideal compensation plan should: 1) provide an incentive for the group's physicians to maintain, or increase, productivity, 2) hold competition amongst the participating doctors (which occurs if compensation is based 100% on productivity) to a minimum, 3) encourage equalization of patient volume (by offering patients the option of seeing other doctors in the group when a requested physician is unavailable), 4) motivate the member physicians to make decisions based on what is best for the group, 5) encourage all doctors to control unnecessary costs, and 6), offer value through participation in the group and, eventually, through partnership.

There are many ways for medical groups to divide income. Let us simplify the options by focusing on four conventional strategies. These can serve as a foundation for creating "hybrids," as necessary, for meeting the unique needs of a specific group. Typical compensation formula categories are based on: 1) individual productivity minus an allocation of total practice expenses, with all doctors contributing an equal amount, 2) equal division of total practice net income, regardless of individual productivity, 3) individual productivity minus overhead for the individual as determined by the practice's overhead percentage, and 4) individual productivity minus overhead for the individual as determined by the practice's overhead percentage, with profit sharing for partners. Each of these formulas has its advantages and disadvantages, depending on the needs of the group.

Productivity Minus Equal Allocation of Total Expenses

This method is most often seen when a group of doctors comes together to practice "under one roof" with the primary goal of sharing expenses and call. In such an arrangement, all common group expenses (such as rent, staff, and supplies) are shared equally, regardless of individual productivity. This arrangement is seldom successful over the long-term because the doctors are not working as a true group and the division of expenses does not adequately meet the five goals to be achieved by an effective compensation formula. When using this format, lower producing doctors end up paying a disproportionate percentage of expenses, making this a much better arrangement for the higher producing ones. A portion of this disparity could be addressed by adjusting the expense allocations to more closely match each doctor's productivity, but the high producing doctors typically perceive this arrangement as being unfair, considering that it's not their "problem" that other doctors in this expense sharing agreement are unable to fully utilize their allocated space and staff. One common exception made by those using this format is accommodation for inequitable billing expenses created by significant differentials in patient volume, by doctor. In this instance, a practice can base billing costs on a percentage of revenue, just as would be done by a billing service. This will reduce total overhead costs for the lower producing doctors and increase it for the more productive ones. Ultimately, an equal expense sharing arrangement is a defensive strategy that is unable to capture the chief opportunities to be gained from practicing in a group.

Equal Division of Total Practice Net Income

I do not see this method being used very often today, but it is an ideal arrangement if the doctors involved see it as being fair. This works best when two or more doctors start a practice together – contributing the same capital, putting in the same hours to build the practice, and each contributing value through his/her own unique interests and skills. This method meets four of the five goals of an ideal compensation formula. Its potential weakness is the fact that it does not provide member doctors with specific incentive to strive for higher individual productivity. This framework does, however, incentivize doctors to be efficient, non-competitive, and share patients. In spite of these advantages, when one doctor in a group becomes ten to fifteen percent more productive than the others and this disparity is ignored, disagreements over the issue of "fairness" tend to develop. Since it is in the entire group's interest for a highly productive doctor to remain so, it is advantageous for every doctor in this "equal salary" arrangement to provide this more productive member with an incentive – such as an additional monthly "guaranteed payment to partner" bonus – for the purpose of acknowledging and encouraging his/her greater contribution.

Productivity Minus Individual Percentage of Overhead

This is the most common format used to determine compensation for doctors who practice in groups, and to a varying degree, it addresses all the five goals of an optimum compensation formula.

If a doctor produces $300,000 in a practice that has a gross profit margin of 40%, the amount available for that doctor's compensation is $120,000 ($300,000 x 40%), with $180,000 going towards overhead ($120,000 x 60%). Compensation for a doctor producing $400,000 would be $160,000 ($400,000 x 40%), with $240,000 going towards overhead ($400,000 x 60%). Doctors who produce more earn more. This method also takes into account the fact that higher producers utilize more of a practice's resources, requiring them to pay a percentage of overhead in proportion to their individual production. The net result is that higher producers earn more and pay a higher portion of overhead.

This method of compensation rewards higher producing doctors with higher pay, while at the same time, enabling lower producing doctors to earn more than they would in a situation in which overhead is split evenly. Such an agreement encourages all doctors to control overhead because this will increase income for every doctor in the group. The one problem with this framework is that it can encourage competition for new patients, and it does not encourage doctors to send their patients to others in the group when they themselves are unavailable.

A variation on this theme would be an allocation of an equal, predetermined percentage of "common overhead" to all doctors in the group, with added individual "cost-centers" to account for any costs created by disproportionate, or exclusive, use of specific resources by specific doctors. For example, one may need the use of more treatment rooms on a regular basis, or s/he may employ an additional nurse who works just with him/her. This doctor would pay a proportionately higher percentage of rent, or the full salary of the "exclusive" staff member. "Perks" that generate these "special" expenses should enable the "user doctors" to be more productive and, therefore, result in greater income for them. This should provide more than enough to offset these doctors' extra contributions to overhead. Some practices take this even further, putting expense items that vary significantly amongst the doctors (such as malpractice or health insurance) into individual doctor "cost centers." At some point, this can be taken to an extreme – with doctors arguing over the allocation of every expense, regardless of how small. When this occurs, a point of diminishing returns is reached at which the time spent determining allocations accomplishes very little other than distracting the participating doctors from the bigger strategic picture – determining how to capture opportunities that will benefit the group as a whole.

Creating an Incentive for Partnership

Ultimately, there is no perfect compensation formula. If all doctors practicing in a group produce within ten percent of each other and all have individual "unquantifiable" contributions to offer, equal salaries work well. If there is a significant gap in individual productivity, a compensation formula based on productivity, minus overhead as determined by the practice's overhead percentage, works well. Ultimately, a hybrid formula of these various methods may be ideal. One such hybrid to consider is to have total compensation be comprised of amounts from multiple sources, such as: 1) a base salary that is fixed for each doctor (which could remain constant, or increase each year, based on the number of years in the practice), 2) a portion of salary based on individual productivity, and 3) a portion based on profit sharing (which could be determined by percentage of ownership). This formula could include additional compensation for doctors who perform group management duties. This would be used to offset any decline in productivity that these doctors may experience as a result of having fewer hours available for rendering patient care.

Such a hybrid provides an incentive for becoming a partner because only partners share in the profit portion of this equation. Establishing a profit pool beyond physicians' salaries also increases the value of a group practice. Profit could come from three potential sources: 1) a small amount withheld from each doctor's revenue, 2) income from ancillaries owned by the group, and 3) contributions from employed associates who are paid a base salary and a lower percentage of productivity than partners. Typically, to qualify for partnership, an associate should be generating enough revenue to fully cover his/her base salary, productivity bonus, and contribution to profit. The amounts of weight given to base salary, productivity, and profit in this "formula" will be different for each group. Ideally, when establishing a compensation formula, you want to optimize both the needs of the individuals and the goals of the group. With the "right" weighting, and periodic "tweaking," your formula can meet all five of the goals of an ideal compensation formula.

Understand Who Today's Buyer Is

Buyers of today's practices, or potential partners in group practices, are likely to be new practitioners, many of whom are already associates of the practices that they are contemplating partnership in or purchase of. The good news is that today's typical graduate is well trained, and new practitioners who are better trained bring potential opportunity to existing practices (especially busy ones whose current owners have good reputations in the community). A hurdle that must be overcome is the fact that associates and owners typically have vastly different perspectives regarding practice value. This, in combination with numerous business and emotional issues that enter the picture throughout the negotiation process, make agreement on value difficult, often resulting in owner/associate breakups. Let us consider a few of these critical issues.

For most medical specialties, the associate is in the driver's seat because demand is greater than supply. If an associate does not become a partner within a few years, s/he has an opportunity to go elsewhere. Two years is a good benchmark figure for assuming that an associate has been in a practice long enough to have made a significant impact. In general, an associate who has been with a practice longer than two years already "owns" a percentage of the practice's goodwill – whether or not the owner is willing to acknowledge this fact. Owners become emotionally biased because they have spent years building their practices and have "given" their associates referral contacts and patients. While this may be the case, it is also true that patient loyalties do change, allowing associates to build their own followings and develop contacts of their own. If buy-in negotiations break down and an associate leaves, patients are free to choose whom they want to see, and a percentage of the practice is going to leave with that associate. Rather than agonizing over this point, it is better to recognize this reality up front and consider its value during the appraisal process.

The longer an associate has been with a practice, the greater is his/her value to that practice. The reality is that after five years, the efforts of an effective associate may have almost doubled a practice's revenue. In such cases, the original owner needs to recognize that s/he has far more to gain financially in the future by working out an affordable partnership with the associate or negotiating reasonable terms for a buy-out.

Both parties in negotiations need to recognize that there is a significant difference between buying into a practice and buying out a partner who is retiring. The majority of a practice's value is its cash flow. In a situation in which a practice is being purchased, or a partner bought-out, the entire cash flow of the owner, or partner, is being acquired, and this could have significant and immediate value. The same does not apply to a buy-in situation in which the value being acquired is primarily one of tangible assets and future opportunity. Because of this, buy-in and buy-out are very different; in a buy-out, the buyer will have access to the cash flow necessary for making larger payments, while the buyer in a buy-in situation rarely does. While every situation differs, allowances need to be made for this reality, and one equitable way to do this is through a reasonable compensation formula.

Valuation focuses solely on the practice, but actual sale price must take into account the financial situation of the buyer. Regardless of a practice's value, or an associate's willingness to pay, student loan payments represent increased risk for a young buyer, and they result in a reduced price for the seller. Most buyers are only able to afford purchases based on what they can afford to pay, per month, and the need to pay student loans decreases this amount. Today, many physicians have incurred student loan debts in excess of $200,000, and it is unlikely that this number will become smaller in the future. Clearly, this will lessen what today's buyers are able to afford.

Numerous business and emotional issues impact the practice valuation and buy-in processes. We have examined only a few of these. Negotiators should not become discouraged; instead, they should be encouraged by studies showing that successful negotiations result in great long-term value for both owners and associates who become partners. Today's associates are enthusiastic, well trained, and bring energy and new skills to a practice – skills which can ignite growth. Statistics show that when all doctors in a practice are partners, they all earn better, and this adds up significantly over the long-term. Creating a successful partnership requires creativity, flexibility, and understanding the sources of a practice's value, and the better that each doctor understands the perspective of the others, the more likely it is that any negotiated buy-in, or buy-out, will work well financially for all parties.

Negotiation Strategies

Whether a practice is being valued for a buy-in, buy-out, practice merger, or sale to a hospital or medical group, a successful outcome is contingent on the participants' ability to negotiate effectively. In fact, the ability to negotiate is important to success in both our business and personal lives. Herb Cohen, author of *You Can Negotiate Anything*, acknowledges the pervasiveness of negotiations in our lives in the following, "Your real world is a giant negotiating table." Negotiating is not just something we do when making major financial transactions (such as taking on an associate, hiring staff, buying equipment, haggling over the terms of a managed care contract, or selling a practice). It also comes into play daily in our offices when discussing procedures or fees with patients and at home where we regularly negotiate with our children or spouses. Because our overall effectiveness in both personal and professional pursuits depends on our negotiating skills, working to improve them should be a lifetime endeavor.

Might reading a book, or two, improve our negotiating skills? Amazon.com lists over 60,000 books on negotiating. *Getting to Yes, Getting Past No, Start With No, Get What You Want, Negotiating With Your Teen, Beyond Winning, Negotiating to Create value in Deals and Disputes, The Power of Nice, Negotiating Rationally, The Negotiation Took Kit,* and *Negotiating for Dummies* are just a few popular titles. Many "negotiation experts," however, believe that books serve little purpose in improving skills and that experience is what really counts. Certainly, authors can provide good examples and clever ways to respond during negotiations, but experts point out that "in the heat of the moment" it is difficult to come up with the clever responses one has seen outlined in a book. I agree that reading books and articles only marginally tends to improve ones skills; however, my analysis of the wide variety of negotiating situations in which I have been personally involved has convinced me that there are several key understandings which can greatly improve a doctor's approach to negotiations and their subsequent outcomes.

Perhaps the greatest challenge to negotiating is that the process generally involves both emotional and economic issues. This complex combination of irrational and rational factors can lead to results which include damaged personal or business relationships and sub-optimal outcomes. In transactions, such as selling a home, the subsequent relationship between the negotiators is irrelevant; however, in others, such as negotiating staff and employed physician salaries, partnership in a medical practice, or working out the details of a third party payer contract, it is critical to future success that a positive relationship is maintained amongst all involved in the negotiations. We want to focus on improving the outcomes for negotiating situations in which both economic and emotional issues are involved and in which maintaining the subsequent relationships amongst the negotiators is important.

There Is Usually a Large Range of Possible Win-Win Outcomes

Participants in negotiations are ideally looking for solutions that will satisfy all parties – "win-win" outcomes. It is important to recognize that there is a wide range of outcomes which will "satisfy" both sides. The proverbial "win-win" does often occur, however, with one side being far more "satisfied" than the other. A good example of this is presented in a classic scene from the movie "Pretty Woman." In this scene, Richard Gere (a wealthy businessman) is negotiating for the services of Julia Roberts (an attractive escort) – to accompany him to various business/social functions. He offers her two thousand dollars for one week of her services, and she counters with an offer of six. He ups his offer to three thousand, and she comes back with five. When he offers four thousand, she agrees, and a deal is struck. After the negotiations are finished, she quickly lets him know that she would have accepted two thousand. He smiles and tells her that he would have paid six – a wide range of outcomes that would have been acceptable to both.

In this example transaction, a win-win "deal" existed anywhere between two and six thousand dollars. We need to recognize that, in most negotiations, there is a similar range of outcomes acceptable to both parties. This emphasizes the importance for a negotiator to include a strategy that identifies as much of this potential range as possible before the negotiation process is begun. If you are capable of discerning this range, your end position in the negotiations is more likely to end up at the high end. Understanding this one concept will make it clear why the subsequent points we will be discussing are so important.

Preparation Should Include Listening

Most of us do not need advice from a book to recognize the importance of adequate preparation for negotiations. Experts point out that thorough preparation is even more important than aggressive argument. Because most of us come into negotiations with a sense that the other side has more information and expertise than we do, we have all the more reason to prepare ourselves. For example, when purchasing a car, we feel at a significant disadvantage because we are not in the auto sales business. If we prepare ahead of time – conducting research to find the amount the dealer paid for the car and, perhaps, the range of prices that our trade-in might command – our own confidence and the outcome of our negotiations will certainly be better.

Not everything can be determined before negotiations are initiated. This is especially true for non-monetary issues, such as determining a person's motivation (beyond price) for wanting a product or service. These important factors can be uncovered only by listening, which is something most people need to work on. One of the most important points made in the book *Getting to Yes* is as follows: "Since the other side will say yes for its reasons, not yours, agreement requires understanding and addressing your counterpart's problem as a means to solving yours." The only way to learn the other side's "reasons" – to determine what it is trying to accomplish – is to listen carefully and ask the right questions.

Since key negotiation issues are both economic and non-economic, there is a wide range of solutions that will result in successful negotiations. For example, an associate looking to affiliate with a practice may have a range of compensation levels s/he is willing to accept because the ultimate dollar amount agreed upon can be balanced out by other non-economic factors, such as work hours, practice location, and/or future opportunities (which might be even more important to him/her than initial compensation). The significance of these factors cannot be given their proper weight without first asking questions and listening carefully to the responses. G. Richard Shell, author of *Bargaining for Advantage*, cites studies showing that the most successful negotiators "happen to be the most persistent question-askers – and listeners." I find it most useful when starting the negotiation process to go in with an open mind and a blank sheet of paper. In this way, I am signaling to the other side that I have no predetermined position and that I am sincerely interested in listening and gaining a better understanding of their interests and ideas.

Understand the Value You Bring to the Table

Know what you have to offer. It is beneficial for you to assess the value that you bring to the table before entering any type of negotiations. Whether you are negotiating to join a group, merge practices, or participate in a managed care contract, it is critical that you understand the economic and non-economic value that you will be bringing to the table.

Determining "value added" is one of the key strategies of game theory, and one way to assess this value is to ask how the future fortunes of the remaining players in the "game" would be affected if you were to leave. This quickly focuses your negotiating strategy on essential issues. Many people tend to over estimate the value they bring to the table and underestimate the value of others. Obviously, this hinders negotiations. A prior self-assessment uncovers the value that you bring to negotiations – which may not be easy to quantify, and it prompts you to improve certain areas – which would enhance your value. If, for example, you lack a specific skill that would increase your value, an effective addition to the negotiation process would be an offer to acquire that skill by a specified date. Knowing clearly ahead of time the value and potential you bring to the table will give you strength in your negotiations.

Know Your Alternatives

In their book, *Getting to Yes*, Roger Fisher, Bill Ury, and Bruce Patton recommend that before entering any negotiations, it is important to determine your BATNA (their acronym for "best alternative to a negotiated agreement"). An economist would refer to this as your "opportunity cost" – your next best alternative or option, should negotiations fail – your fallback position. When making any type of economic decision, your ultimate value is determined by your next best option, which is the opportunity you must forego in order to pursue your chosen path.

Knowing your opportunity cost – the proverbial "bottom line" – protects you from accepting any agreement you should reject and helps you reach an agreement that satisfies as many of your interests as possible. Both sides involved in negotiations have opportunity costs. We can safely assume that whomever we are negotiating with also has a bottom line, and one of the focuses of negotiations should be to identify this limiting boundary. The concept of putting oneself in another's shoes may be old, but it is irreplaceable. It is important that you know your counterpart's opportunity costs – what s/he desires, or needs, from negotiations.

Letting Them Have Your Way

The ultimate outcome to be achieved from any negotiation process is for the other side to come up with the suggestion of exactly what it is you want. The better you understand your counterpart's needs (the more carefully you listen), the more likely it is that you will be able to articulate a logical path which will lead him/her to "come up with" suggestions which meet your needs. Obviously, if the other side proposes what you want, a successful implementation is virtually assured, and your relationship is strengthened in the process. Since the success of a business depends on good working relationships, this is the most productive form of negotiating possible, and it facilitates the pursuit of future mutual opportunities.

In an April 2001 *Harvard Business Review* article entitled "Six Habits of Merely Effective Negotiators," James K. Sebenius quoted the Italian Diplomat, Daniele Vare, as saying, "Negotiation is the art of letting them have your way." He also gave the example of Francois de Callieres, an eighteenth-century commentator, who stated, "Negotiation masters possess the supreme art of making every man offer him as a gift that which it was his chief design to secure." The better you are at listening and finding ways to solve the problems of the "other side," the more likely you are to obtain this sort of result from your negotiations.

Focus on Interests, Not Positions

One of the most significant distinctions made in the book, *Getting to Yes,* is of the difference that exists between interests and positions. A *position* is defined as something that you have decided upon while *interests* are what caused you to so decide. There are usually multiple positions capable of satisfying any given interest. People often enter negotiations having already decided on a position that will only serve to slow or block the process. Since the goal of all negotiations is to satisfy collective interests, it is important to begin with an open mind and focus on interests rather than on positions.

Even when the interests of two parties are quite different, they may be complimentary. For example, a doctor and a potential associate may hold different and incompatible *positions* regarding the first year's salary; however, if they enter into negotiations which focus on interests, rather than on positions, the doctors are likely to find a solution to the issue of salary since most interests in this type of negotiation are usually compatible (i.e. both want the practice to grow and prosper). A focus on common interests is likely to stimulate both sides to find mutually beneficial solutions. Even though salary can be a difficult issue, a focus on the skills, attributes, and attitudes that a new associate will bring to a practice should make salary less of a roadblock in negotiations. The associate should be prepared to demonstrate the ways s/he will contribute that will support his/her desired salary (such as increasing productivity for the owner while reducing his/her current workload).

Negotiations are seldom one-shot, single-issue deals. More typically, they are spread over an extended period of time and are complex, include multiple relationships, and involve both economic and non-economic issues. One of my favorite *Harvard Business Review* cartoons illustrating failed negotiations depicts a group of despondent business people assembled around a conference table with the following caption: "The key difference with the new plan is that what we once feared most is now our best case scenario." To avoid this type of outcome for your negotiations, it is critical that you understand the importance of the following: 1) preparing thoroughly, 2) identifying the range of mutually acceptable outcomes, 3) understanding your value, 4) knowing your options, 5) listening carefully, and 6) focusing on mutual interests in order to find solutions that will enable each side to "have its way." Ultimately, we get what we negotiate.

Chapter 11

Be Smarter with Your Money

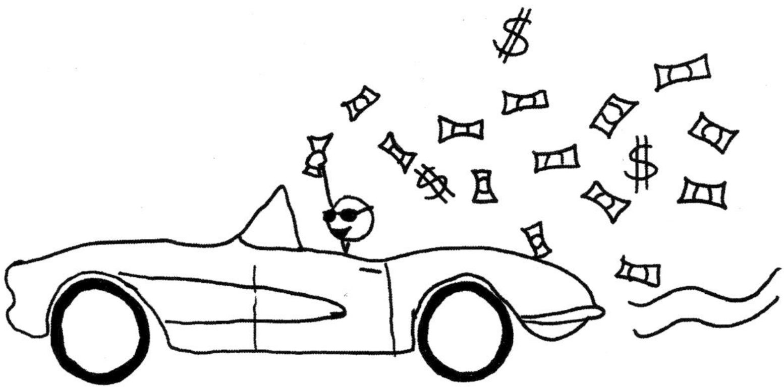

Achieving Financial Independence

Financial independence is a basic goal for most of us. This goal is as important to someone who plans to continue working part-time indefinitely because s/he enjoys work as it is to someone who wants to, someday, retire completely. Achieving financial independence has always been difficult, but it is becoming ever more so. Many who seemed to be on track have seen their net worth decline substantially in recent years. We have also seen those in the business of giving financial advice fall on hard times. If these "experts" don't have all the answers, what chance do the rest of us have?

When we look at the long-term road to financial independence, we realize that the basics have not really changed and that every working person does have a good chance of achieving this goal. If anything, the events of recent years should reinforce the value of developing good financial habits, exercising discipline, and applying common sense to financial decisions. If you were to choose just one financial habit that you absolutely should follow, it would be: "pay yourself first." Regardless of your income level or stage of practice, the first "bill" that you pay each month should be to *yourself*; as your income increases, you will never miss this money. It has been shown that, without this discipline, many high earners never achieve financial independence.

The old "rule of thumb" for becoming financially independent was to save ten percent of pre-tax income each year and aim for growing the principal ten percent each year. This formula, over a twenty-five year period, would result in a nest egg that (along with Social Security) would return the same retirement income as that which a person had earned during his/her final year of employment. In spite of the fact that this approach once virtually "guaranteed" financial independence at the time of retirement, few actually reached this goal, even in good economic times. The average annual savings rate in the U.S. fluctuates, often falling well below ten percent. Making matters even worse, achieving consistent annual investment returns of ten percent, or higher, is riskier and more difficult to count on today. One saving grace at present is that people are living longer and healthier lives. This allows more options when determining when to retire or whether to plan on working part-time during "retirement." There are no easy solutions to achieving financial independence, but unless your plan is to win the lottery, or you happen to have very wealthy relatives, you need to put a plan into place through which you will be able to achieve this goal.

An alternative "rule of thumb" (if you if you plan to fully retire at age 65, at 80% of your pre-retirement earnings) is that you will need a nest egg of approximately twelve times your income, in addition to Social Security. To determine if you are on track for meeting this goal, Charles Farrell, author of *Your Money Ratios: 8 Simple Tools for Financial Security*, recommends that by age 35, you should have accumulated a savings of 1.4 times your salary. This ratio increases to 3.7 at age 45, and to 7.1 at 55. These outcomes assume that you are investing 12% to 15% of your salary and are earning 4.5 percentage points above inflation each year. Depending on your age, and how closely you are hitting these milestones, you have the option of adjusting your savings rate and/or retirement date accordingly.

The Path to Your First $1,000,000

Setting personal financial goals is an important step in reaching financial independence. The first step in this process is to ask the question, "How much money will be enough?" Will Rogers responded to this question with, "Just a little bit more." A *cnnmoney.com* poll conducted in February of 2010 asked, "How much money would you need to feel secure?" Twelve percent responded with, "$500,000," eighteen percent said, "$500,000 to $1 million," thirty two percent said "$1 million to $2 million," and thirty eight percent said, "more than $2 million." There is no universally agreed upon answer to this question, but one benchmark commonly used for measuring wealth is a million dollars. While I am not suggesting a million dollars as *the goal* for achieving financial independence, simply knowing the amount of time you would need to reach $1 million in savings and investments will help you to set in place a realistic plan and timeline for reaching your goal. If your next goal is to continue growing this nest egg towards multi-million dollar levels, having this first million to invest while you are still working is going to make your goal more easily achievable.

While most Americans would like to be millionaires, according to the research firm, Spectrem Group, as of 2011, fewer than seven per cent of households in the U.S. actually were. In a *USA Today* cover story entitled, "Everyone Wants a Shot at being a Millionaire," analyst Danny Sheridan attempted to calculate the odds of accumulating one million dollars over thirty years, using various strategies. His results are depicted in *Table 11.1*:

Table 11.1: Odds of Accumulating $1,000,000 Over 30 Years

Strategy	Odds of making $1,000,000
Owning a small business	1 in 1,000
Working for a dot-com that goes public	1 in 10,000
Saving $800 a month for 30 years @ 7.1% return	1 in 1.5 million
Winning a game show	1 in 4 million
Playing the slots in a casino	1 in 6 million
Winning the lottery	1 in 12 million
Inheriting $1,000,000	1 in 12 million

I would expect that the odds against winning a million dollars would be very high; however, what shocked me the most amongst Sheridan's calculations is that only one person in 1.5 million becomes a millionaire using the strategy of investing $800 a month, at 7.1%, for thirty years. Of all the possibilities he considered, this is the only one that guarantees attainment of one million dollars; yet, according to his research, only one person in one and a half million actually applies this strategy!

Saving, investing, and risk are at the heart of all financial plans. What has changed since Sheridan's 2000 survey is that 1) achieving financial independence will require saving more than ten percent of pre-tax income each year, and 2) because returns on investment now fluctuate more dramatically from year to year, it is likely that it will require more than twenty five years to achieve this goal. You will need a *Plan B* in place just in case you fall short of your goal and need to work part-time in order to augment this income.

As daunting as the task of achieving financial independence may seem, a good way to start on the road to attaining it is to estimate the annual income you believe you will need in retirement and work backwards from that point to determine the amount you must invest each year in order to achieve a nest egg of sufficient size to deliver this amount annually. By quantifying your end goal, you will have a better idea of how much you need to put away each year, what your annual return needs to be, and how many years this will take.

As each year passes, you will be able to reassess your progress and determine whether to adjust your savings rate, your time frame, your desired retirement lifestyle, or your need to continue working part-time during "retirement." If you "get lucky" along the way and achieve a higher than expected rate of return, you will simply achieve your goal sooner – or have a larger nest egg at your predetermined retirement age; however, without a plan in place, even if you are a high earner, you still may not achieve financial independence at the point in time you had planned.

Starting at your goal and working backwards to determine the steps needed to reach that goal is consistent with Steven Covey's "second habit" (found in his book *The Seven Habits of Highly Effective People*). This is the habit of "beginning with the end in mind." To see how this approach will point you in the right direction when developing a plan, assume that the financial independence target for maintaining your current lifestyle in retirement is an income of $150,000 a year. If you would like to keep the principal of your nest egg intact, you can make the assumption that this goal would require a nest egg of $2,142,842, yielding 7%, annually. If you are thirty years old and want to be financially independent at age sixty, you would calculate that with a conservative estimated annual growth rate of 7%, you would need to save $22,685 a year in order to achieve this goal. This is valuable information to start with.

What do you do, now that you have this "end point" information? For starters, if you are not now saving this amount, you know that you need to do one or more of the following: 1) reduce the size of your target nest egg and, therefore, the lifestyle you had hoped for at retirement, 2) increase your savings rate, 3) plan on working to an older age, or working part-time in retirement, 4) change your investment philosophy to one that might require taking greater risk, or 5) at retirement, plan on depleting the principal of your nest egg at a rate at which it will, hopefully, last longer than you do.

If you decide to reduce the size of the nest egg that you will have in place at retirement, part of your plan should be to determine the best options for places where you can retire on less money. Financial journals and organizations such as AARP publish articles each year researching the best places to retire – focusing primarily on life-style, cost of living, and access to quality healthcare.

Choosing to increase your savings rate will take discipline and require that you and your spouse agree on the necessary tradeoffs between the needs of today and those of tomorrow. Since we cannot always have everything we want, every financial decision requires that we set priorities and make tradeoffs. If your plan had been to retire at age sixty, changing that plan to working five years longer would allow you to reduce the annual savings requirement (in this case, from $22,685 a year down to $15,402) necessary for achieving the same size nest egg. With ever-increasing healthy life expectancies, working beyond retirement age, especially part-time, has become a popular option because it reduces the amount of savings and/or number of years required for "retirement." More importantly, many people enjoy staying involved with their work, especially on a reduced work schedule.

Your most uncertain choice is to invest the $22,685 in a riskier investment, hoping to hit the historic stock market average return of ten percent, or higher. Over thirty years, at ten percent growth, your nest egg would grow to more than $3,700,000 – giving you even greater security than you had originally planned for; or, if you so chose, you could retire at a younger age because, at a 10% earnings rate, you would hit your original $2,142,842 goal much sooner than planned. In general, it is better to estimate conservatively. If you do end up achieving a higher than 7%

return, you can adjust your financial plan going forward to reflect this greater growth rate; you will become financially independent sooner.

I have heard many reasons from doctors who earn good incomes as to why they continue putting off "paying themselves first." Regardless of what the economy looks like today, we know that over the next thirty years, there will be times when it is booming and others when it is in recession. If you are always paying yourself first, the fluctuating economy will have little impact on your ability to ultimately reach financial independence.

Investment Strategies

Will Rogers once said, "It's not what we don't know that gets us in trouble, it's what we know that isn't so." When it comes to reaching our investment goals, both "what we don't know" and "what we know that isn't so" can get us in trouble. Doctors work hard for their money and any that remains after paying bills and providing for family needs should be made to work equally hard for them.

All investors have the same goal: earn the highest possible return with the least amount of risk. This winning strategy sounds simple, but few investors achieve it – including the "experts." Reward is in proportion to risk, and the challenge is to reduce risk without reducing reward. Generally speaking, the greater a strategy's potential return, the greater its risks. *Table 11.2* shows the payout to be gained from investing $10,000, annually, at various rates of return, over a 36-year period.

This chart makes it clear that the sooner you start investing, the better. It also illustrates the extreme variance in results, depending on the rate of return, length of the time horizon, and investment style. By historic stock market standards, achieving a 12% annual rate of return over a thirty-year time horizon has not been big a stretch. If we were to look at the 32-year period between 1965 and 1997, the S&P 500 average rate of return was 12.9%. One could even have achieved a higher rate if s/he had happened to select the "right" stocks. Of course, many strategies can beat the market in any given year, but few do so consistently. Certainly, if your goal is to become financially independent, your strategy should not be dependent on consistently "beating the market."

Table 11.2: Time Value of Money

Dollar Amount	Rate	$s in 12 years	$s in 18 years	$s in 24 years	$s in 30 years	$s in 36 years
10,000	4%	150,258	256,454	390,826	560,849	775,983
10,000	5%	159,171	281,324	445,020	664,388	958,363
10,000	6%	168,699	309,057	508,156	790,581	1,191,209
10,000	7%	178,885	339,990	581,767	944,607	1,489,134
10,000	8%	189,771	374,502	667,648	1,132,832	1,871,021
10,000	9%	201,407	413,013	767,898	1,363,075	2,361,247
10,000	10%	213,843	455,992	884,973	1,644,940	2,991,268
10,000	11%	227,132	503,959	1,021,742	1,990,209	3,801,644
10,000	12%	241,331	557,497	1,181,552	2,413,327	4,844,631

Warren Buffet is one name that comes to many people's minds when they think of "beating the market." Between these same years – 1965 to 1997 – his average rate of return was a whopping 24.9%! Had our sample $10,000 annual investment grown at this rate, it would have grown to over $120 million by the end of our 36-year time horizon. I have mentioned Warren Buffett from time to time because there is something useful that can be learned from his investment strategy, something which can help physicians when making investment decisions. Buffet's strategy is particularly amazing considering that he used an investment style considered "less risky". During the time that he was consistently achieving the highest growth rate in the stock market, he actually was also taking on the least amount of risk possible; the standard deviation of Buffet's stock portfolio was 13, while the S&P 500's was 16.4. By *definition*, Buffett's strategy was less risky!

It is important to your financial future that you understand the investment style that Buffett employed in earning such a high rate of return while taking on the least amount of risk. This is especially helpful for doctors whose education includes much of the same basic scientific knowledge that Buffett himself uses to beat market averages. In spite of the tremendous amount of relevant knowledge that doctors actually possess, most fail to achieve consistent, above average returns because they use investment styles that work against their long-term investment goals. They can rectify this problem if they understand how Buffett's investment style contradicts much conventional wisdom. Doctors must recognize those areas where "what they know, may not be so."

Few people have the courage or patience to stay with consistent, long-term, investments – especially in the face of short-term market fluctuations and constant bombardment from media and friends hyping the latest "hot stock" or investment fad. Since investment style has a major impact on long-term performance, it is important to understand which styles are doomed to long-term failure and which virtually "guarantee" success. The most common investment styles could be called: 1) the "safe" investor, 2) the "gambler," 3) the "trusting" investor, 4) the "shotgun" investor, and 5) the "focused, smart" investor.

The Safe Investor:

The safe investor fears taking any type of risk with his/her hard earned money. S/he is content to earn a *guaranteed low rate of return* in exchange for peace of mind. Safe, low-yield savings and money market accounts are an essential part of financial planning, but they should not be considered investments. They are ways to "park" money that might be needed for meeting short-term expenses or emergencies. Safe investors tend to "invest" in whole life insurance policies. They are willing to tolerate low returns, accepting the argument that an insurance policy is a form of forced savings. Presumably, these investors accept their agents' rationale that they are not disciplined enough to save money and make their own smart investment decisions.

Savings accounts are "risk-free" because: 1) the principal does not fluctuate, 2) they are insured against loss, and 3) the rate of return is "guaranteed." Since the rate of return for a savings account typically is barely above the rate of inflation, these "risk-free" accounts also guarantee that they will never help anyone achieve financial security. Most "experts" recommend keeping at least six months' income in a safe account; I disagree. This is unrealistic in the early years of family life – especially when paying education costs, and it works against early investment in one's career. Financial planners argue that this "safe" money is needed for emergencies such as a losing a job. This is not applicable to most doctors for whom job security is virtually assured and access to a line of credit could serve the same purpose as cash put away for an emergency.

The "Gambler"

Most people who consider themselves investors are really stock market "gamblers" and just don't know it. They truly believe they are investing. The difference between gambling and investing can be explained in terms of expectations. A gambler is risking money (money that might be needed to meet financial obligations in the short term) with the expectation of making a short-term gain greater than the risk-free rate of return (the rate paid by a short-term, bank CD). Lottery players expect to put down a small amount of money and become instant millionaires. Stock market gamblers put down larger sums and expect similar results. Over the long term, the chances of a gambling investor "winning" are not much better than those for someone playing the lottery. Because these investors can always point to a few winners, they stick with this strategy.

Stock market gambling includes strategies such as day trading, timing the market, investing in "hot tips" – companies expected to become the next Microsoft or IBM, commodity trading, panic selling during market downturns, buying on margin, selling short, and the list goes on. We all know that we can sometimes beat the odds over the short-term; however, the longer our time horizon, the greater the probability that the odds will catch up with us. Investors with relevant knowledge can use the same statistical odds to their advantage – virtually "guaranteeing" them a win over the long term.

Warren Buffet addresses the issue of the gambling investor with the following: "If you're an investor, you're looking at what the asset – in our case, businesses – will do. If you're a speculator, you're primarily forecasting on what the price will do, independent of the business." The odds of predicting whether share prices will be up or down over a short period of time are the same as the odds of predicting the toss of a coin. You will win and lose along the way, but eventually you will end up breaking even. This means that your lifetime total return will be zero (assuming that the gambler doesn't compensate for poor returns by constantly increasing the size of the bet).

Using a different investment style and extending your time line out, even a few years, dramatically lowers this risk. From what I have learned from studying numerous financial theories, I can assure you that these tools may be useful for predicting short-term price and market movements, independent of a specific business, but they will not help an investor achieve above average returns over the long-term. There is no question that the best day traders can make money predicting price movements, independent of the underlying businesses, but this takes a great deal of knowledge and a full-time focus. Even then, very smart people can still lose their shirts. Since prices do track a business over the long-term, why not go for a sure thing?

One of the more "controversial" things I have ever done was to fund a pension plan with borrowed money. With four children and private school payments, I could envision no point in time at which I felt I would have "extra" money to invest. Don't confuse this strategy with the "gambler" who buys stocks on margin – where a margin call during a down market can force the sale of a stock (a time when we should be buying more). I had been looking to buy a new car, and my reasoning was that if I felt I could make payments on a car that was guaranteed to be worth almost nothing in ten years, I could, instead, afford to keep my old car and make those same "car payments" on an investment that should grow over the next ten years. What were the odds that I could build a portfolio of companies whose total worth would be worth less than my intended car purchase after ten years?

Instead of buying this new car, I borrowed $20,000 and opened a Keogh plan. Six months later, instead of driving a recent model car that already would have depreciated thousands of dollars, I received an income tax refund of $6,850 (because of my tax sheltered investment), and I owned ten growing companies – soon worth more than the car. Had I listened to the "experts," I still would have been building my initial Keogh plan years later. I was able to start my plan six years sooner, and by using the appropriate investment style for managing this portfolio, it has turned out that I was able to reduce the size of my future contributions in years when the financial demands of educating four children took precedence.

The "Trusting" Investor

"Trusting" investors feel that stockbrokers, money managers, and mutual fund managers have the ability to make better investment decisions than they can. They also naively trust that these professionals have their customers' best interests at heart. In the case of brokers, the odds are that they have neither. One obvious reason for this is that the commission system establishes an inherent conflict of interests for brokers; the more trades they make, the more money they earn. Also, what about the competency of these advisors? According to Warren Buffett, the Cambridge Group found that 40% of brokers are inexperienced and under-trained.

Most "small" investors purchase shares in mutual funds in order to procure the skills of professional money managers and reduce risk by owning a large variety of stocks. Is this really the best way to invest? Professionally managed U.S. stock funds rarely beat the return of the market as a whole over the long term, and many often do worse than the market average. For the entire year of 1998, the S&P 500 increased 28.6%, yet 20% of all U.S. equity funds lost money that same year!

Mutual funds pay huge salaries because their managers are expected to beat market indexes, but in 1998, only 17% of fund managers actually beat those indexes. If we extend this time horizon beyond five years, fewer than 10% of fund managers beat those indexes. Because so few funds actually beat market indexes, most "experts" are now recommending that investors put their money in index funds (funds that invest in all 30 stocks of the Dow Jones Industrial Index or all 500 of the S&P 500 stocks). *Table 11.3* compares the average fund result with several market indexes over a ten-year period.

Table 11.3: Ten Year Average Returns

Investment Objective	1988 – 1998 Average Annual Return
DJIA	+18.78%
S&P 500	+18.97%
Small company index fund	+7.71%
Average Stock Fund	+14.87%
Average Bond Fund	+8.24%

For those who have no desire to manage money, or actually believe they lack the time to do so, the Dow Jones Industrial index, or the S&P 500, appears to be a good choice.

The "Shotgun" Investor

The "shotgun" investor does a little of everything, with the hope that making some of the right moves will eventually create wealth. These "moves" might include: owning shares in mutual funds, buying individual stocks based on tips, buying "extra" stocks to diversify, buying gold, buying bonds, selling stocks short, purchasing real estate, or trying any other idea that might come into vogue. Diversification is at the heart of this strategy.

Every business school and financial expert teaches diversification as the appropriate way to reduce risk. Everyone agrees with the statement, "Don't put all your eggs in one basket," but what is the optimum number of "baskets"? Since investment risk is defined as the degree of price fluctuation, diversifying a portfolio by adding stocks will reduce risk because it reduces, or smoothes, price fluctuations. Price fluctuations are only a short-term risk, however, and they tend to even out over the long term. Statistically, it has been determined that to obtain the optimum risk reduction from diversifying a portfolio, that portfolio should contain between ten and fifteen stocks. While prices do not necessarily track earnings' growth over the short-term, they typically do over the long-term. It is critical for an investor to understand that too much diversification will actually reduce the long-term, total return of his/her portfolio!

The treatise *Art of War* (conceived by Sun Tzu) refers to preparing for an enemy attack during war, "If I prepare everywhere – I will be weak everywhere." The shotgun approach is like this; it is unfocused – making it weak everywhere.

The Focused, "Smart" Investor

My introduction to the stock market was in 1972 when I became acquainted with a money manager. This friend later went on to start several mutual funds. Early in his career, he analyzed companies one at a time and made personal visits to each of them, interviewing and evaluating management. He knew that if he understood an industry, its product or service, and the company financials, what he was really investing in was management. One of the companies he liked at that time was Wal-Mart, explaining to me that he was not investing in Wal-Mart but was, instead, investing in its founder and manager, Sam Walton. He told me that if the economy or markets changed, a stock price might drop, but a good manager would figure out what to do sooner than his/her competitors, and his/her company's stock price would eventually recover. He felt that Sam Walton was just such a manager. My friend invested in Wal-Mart early and stayed with Sam for a long time.

The first two years of our friendship, 1972 – 1974, happened to be the worst two-year market history of the time; yet, this money manager was upbeat and unconcerned about the daily and yearly market fluctuations. He knew that this simply presented him with the opportunity to increase his investments in companies he already liked. I was just starting practice at the time and, unfortunately, felt that I had no money to invest. My experience with him, however, set much of the foundation for my later investment style.

In 1973, this same money manager told me that I should consider investing in Berkshire Hathaway. This was my first introduction to Warren Buffett, the investment manager for Berkshire Hathaway. Unfortunately, I thought I couldn't afford to buy even one share of that stock at the time (I'm guessing it was around $400 which, to me, sounded high for one share of stock), but at that same time, I borrowed money to purchase a new Volvo station wagon, which cost me $4,800. Today (2011), one share of that same stock sells for $125,599 (the stock never split). What if I, instead, had "sacrificed" and bought a used Volvo, in good condition, and invested $2,000 in Berkshire Hathaway? Well, you can do the math and find out how very expensive my new Volvo actually was.

Warren Buffet believes that an investor captures the best returns and is exposed to the lowest risk if s/he focuses investments in only a few companies – certainly in no more than ten. He states, "With each investment you make, you should have the courage and the conviction to place at least ten percent of your net worth in that stock." Buffet spends his time analyzing the economics of the underlying business and assessing its management, rather than analyzing price movements. He is patient, and his annual stock turnover rate is less than twenty percent. Compare this with most mutual funds that may be composed of hundreds of stocks and often have turnover rates greater than 100%. Mutual fund managers don't tend to manage their funds using the same buy and hold philosophy that they recommend for their investors, and their long-term returns reflect the fact that too much diversification and high turnover can actually reduce yield. If you don't believe me, compare the historical results of the thousands of funds to those achieved by Buffett.

Granted, the average investor does not have the exceptional stock selection abilities of Warren Buffet, but I contend that the average doctor has as many, or more, of these abilities than the typical stockbroker or mutual fund manager. To quote Buffett, "Becoming a successful investor requires a multidisciplinary approach to your thinking. That approach puts you in a different place from almost everyone else because the world is not multidiscipline. Business professors typically don't include physics in their lectures, physics teachers don't include biology, biology teachers don't include mathematics, and mathematicians rarely include psychology in their coursework." The reality is that a doctor's training is multidisciplinary, and doctors who manage private practices understand most relevant management principles. What they need to do is unlearn most of the financial misinformation they have heard and read.

Buffet points out that if you look closely at the words and actions of a company's management team, you will find clues for measuring the value of their work long before it shows up in financial reports or the stock pages. Review a company's annual reports from the past few years, and see what management has said about future strategies. Compare this to what they have actually done. In addition to understanding business operations, analysis of most companies requires only simple algebra, basic probability theory, and an understanding of strategy. The best strategy comes from understanding games, and Buffett has been a passionate bridge player since college. He sees parallels between the game of bridge and investing because, "Bridge is a game of a million inferences, you're seeing through new situations every ten minutes, it is about weighing gain/loss ratios, and you're doing calculations all the time." Business is about strategy, and in business, you are not competing against other companies, but against the strategy of other companies' management teams. This "game" style of thinking can be used to evaluate these companies.

Where to Start

You should begin by continuing what you are already doing. Don't sell your mutual funds; hold on to the stocks you already own, and don't fire your broker just yet. If you have no investments, it's time to start – even if you have to borrow the money. You're never too old, or too young, to begin. My son even owned stocks when he was eleven years old. You are going to need this skill throughout your lifetime, and now is the time to get on the learning curve. Don't think of this as work because it actually becomes fun. Begin by studying companies and their industries, reading their reports, following what management says, and studying the strategies of other companies in the same industries. Stick to what you know.

There are thousands of companies out there, and you only need to own a few (between five and fifteen). Don't buy everything at once. You may buy only one stock to start. If you already own stocks, you may benefit most by analyzing the companies you currently hold and then selling a few. The next company you buy should be better than the ones you already own. Why add a company to your portfolio that is not as good as the ones you already own simply for the sake of diversification? This will only serve to lower your long-range earnings. Follow the companies you do own very closely – this is easier when you own only a few and have access to on-line research and information. Don't pay attention to daily market fluctuations, unless there is a big drop in the entire market – which will enable you to pick up cheaper shares of the companies you are already following.

You do not need to add industries you don't understand – or companies with products or services you don't understand – simply for diversification's sake. Warren Buffett is a close friend of Bill Gates (Microsoft CEO) and Andy Grove (Intel CEO), but he achieved his high returns without owning their companies or any of the "high flying" technology or healthcare stocks of the nineties. He avoids these industries because he says that he does not understand them. What are the odds you won't be able to find and maintain a portfolio of ten good companies that are capable of achieving average, or possibly above average returns for the next ten, twenty, or thirty years in the industries that you *do* understand? Remember, you can make many bad choices along the way and still become financially independent. Even Warren Buffett drops 20% of his companies each year. If you are following the companies you hold and understand the industries they are in, you will know if a time comes when management is no longer responding to market needs.

There is no financial "law" that requires you to own something from every major industry. Interestingly, over the years, some of the best stocks have been healthcare related. This is a good place to start your research since it is a field you are familiar with. Healthcare is a huge industry, with such diverse areas as pharmaceuticals, hospitals, home health care, HMOs, nursing homes, surgery centers, medical products, medical software, medical supplies, and biomedical products and research. In an industry that we understand well, we should know long before the "experts" when it is time to buy or sell.

Even if you make a bad choice and experience a significant drop in stock price before you sell a company to replace it with a better one, your long-term results will hardly be affected. What if you select ten bad companies? This is highly unlikely, but this is why I suggest that you, initially, keep a third of your investments in your best performing funds and some cash in safe, high yielding interest vehicles. Over time, your portfolio weightings will increase in the areas in which you are doing better simply because you will not be selling off these good stocks.

Don't Be Tempted to Day-Trade

Financial independence should be the primary objective of your financial plan. To achieve this independence requires not only that you make a good income, but also that you live within your means and regularly invest a portion of your income, allowing sufficient time for it to grow. Most often, such a plan has a thirty to forty year time horizon unless, of course, you happen to "get lucky" along the way. There are numerous investment styles, but in most cases, it is the slow, steady, buy-and-hold investor who wins the race. While you will encounter day traders and market timers who claim to have accumulated great wealth, the odds of winning with this strategy are against you, and even if you are inclined to try it, the time, attention, knowledge, and experience required to engage in this kind of investing leave little time for practicing medicine.

Consider a study of 66,000 investors in which it was found that, of this group, those who traded most frequently earned seven percentage points a year less than those who were the least active traders. A seven percent gap is almost insurmountable. A handicap of even one or two percent, compounded over a period of thirty years, can change results from spectacular to average. For example, if you invest $1,000, annually, and achieve an average return of ten percent a year, at the end of forty years, you will have a total investment of $4,425,000. If these earnings drop by just one percent annually, this amount lowers by more than $1,000,000. Normally, stock trades should be made for the purpose of taking some profit from a company that has had a significant increase in price, or for the purpose of dropping a company that no longer meets your original criteria for buying it. When it comes to effective stock trading, for most people, the "rule" for frequency of trades should be, "less is more."

The same "less is more" policy applies to a medical practice. When seeking strategies to make a practice more profitable, the default option for most doctors is to focus on finding ways of increasing volume. Sometimes, this is necessary, but at others, it is not. Don't just go to "default" when making decisions. When strategizing, always consider the possibility that less might be more.

The Invisible Risk to Your Nest Egg

Planning for retirement is an important element of every physician's financial strategy. To avoid the damage that could result from a mistake being made – and then compounded – over a thirty-year period, many employ the services of professional planners. These physicians are looking to avoid risks that could cause them to fall short of their goals. In spite of the professional advice they receive, I find that the investment strategies being employed by many doctors accomplish the exact opposite of what they are trying to achieve – exposing them to great financial risk in retirement. As you will see, "risk" can come from where you least expect it.

Let us take a look at four possible scenarios faced by a doctor at sixty five, the typical target age for retirement: 1) s/he may not live to sixty five, 2) s/he may live only a few years beyond sixty five, 3) s/he may become disabled, with the worst case scenario being the development of an incapacitating mental disability such as Alzheimer's or dementia, or 4) s/he may live a long and healthy life. Of these four possibilities, only the fourth presents a retiree with significant financial risk. Imagine a long and healthy life being the worst-case financial scenario! While the first two possibilities are certainly undesirable, neither presents significant financial risk because, under either of these circumstances, the doctor is unlikely to outlive his/her financial resources. To protect a surviving spouse, however, a financial plan should include life and disability insurance. The third risk can be addressed through the purchase of long-term care insurance.

Given that outliving one's money is the greatest "risk" to be addressed when devising a financial plan, let us look at two serious mistakes that, if avoided, can help us decrease this risk. The first, made by many physicians strategizing for retirement, is being too conservative and protective of invested capital. This is especially evident following years in which both the real estate and stock markets have taken large hits. While an extremely conservative investment approach might guarantee that a plan will not lose principal in any given year, it also virtually *guarantees* that the investment's growth rate will be insufficient to build resources great enough to protect against the "risk" of living a long and healthy life. The outcome of "extreme protection" is that the doctor will probably need to continue working for more years than s/he had planned.

As an example, assume that a practitioner takes home $150,000 yearly, sets aside $30,000 each year in a retirement account (starting at age 35), and retires at 65. If this money is placed in "safe" investments, it might return about 4% a year, and if the doctor continues this strategy until age 65, his/her portfolio will be worth about $1.7 million at "retirement." Withdrawing 4% a year from this account in retirement years (the amount recommended by most financial planners) would generate an annual income of $67,000. If, instead, this same amount had been invested in a diversified stock portfolio that earned an average annual return rate of 8%, 10%, or 12%, the portfolio value at age 65 would reach, approximately $3.4 million, $4.9 million, or $7.2 million, respectively – producing an annual incomes (at the same 4% withdrawal rate) of $136,000, $196,000 or $290,000. When we include the additional money the doctor will receive from social security, even the 8% return would fully replace his/her current income. This "riskier" strategy protects against inflation because the portfolio is growing at a faster rate than the rate of withdrawal. Equally important, if the doctor desires, the annual income s/he withdraws at retirement could be much higher because portfolios of this size are unlikely to be depleted, even when withdrawing percentages of more than 4% a year.

The stock market has had its ups and downs over the years; yet, depending on which index you follow, it has historically yielded a 10% to 12% average annual rate of return. While this level of return is not "guaranteed," the odds that this rate will average less than 4% over the next 35 years are low. In this unlikely event, it really would not matter whether one had invested "safely" (protecting principal) or "smartly" (investing principal at an acceptable level of risk), because the outcome of either strategy would be the same – in order to generate enough income, the doctor would need to continue working beyond his/her projected retirement age. This being the case, the two strategies have the same downside – a downside that is *guaranteed* when using the "safe" strategy but highly unlikely with the "risky" strategy. What is significant is that only the "risky" strategy has the potential upside of providing financial security, regardless of how many years one lives.

Based on the outcomes of the two scenarios discussed above, the possibility of working past sixty-five should be an integral part of anyone's financial plan. As part of this strategy, when a physician approaches the age at which s/he is considering the sale of a practice, s/he should consider including a clause which allows the option of continuing to work in the practice (at least part-time) following the sale. While this might reduce the sale price, this option is "priceless" should it ever be needed – whether for personal or financial reasons. Fortunately, if we are lucky enough to be healthy and live well beyond the age of sixty-five, we will, by definition, also have the option of, and ability to, continue working. Keeping this option open is a way to reduce the risks associated with longevity and/or inflation – with more assurance that our money will "last" as long as we do.

The opportunity to work part time as an "employee" upon sale of one's practice allows a physician the opportunity to shed the responsibility of management and reduce his/her hours to the point of being "semi-retired." This offers the best of both worlds – especially to the doctor for whom full retirement turns out to be less fulfilling than envisioned. How much is this option worth? Consider that a doctor working two days a week in a busy practice should be able to produce a "take home salary" of at least $80,000, even if s/he no longer performs surgery. For the conservative investor, this $80,000 annual income is the equivalent of the earnings that would be produced by a $1.6 million nest egg.

Not only doctors "fear longevity," and enterprising companies are creating products that capitalize on this fear. A few insurers have introduced "longevity insurance." In some cases, purchasing insurance to protect against the possibility of outliving a nest egg makes sense; yet, according to Shane Chalke, CEO of Seven Squared Financial, in an article from the July 16, 2007, issue of *BusinessWeek*, entitled "More Dollars Later in Life," "What you are really buying with such policies is the freedom to spend a greater percentage of your savings in retirement than would otherwise be prudent – some 7% a year, versus 4% – knowing that this safety net will fall into place."

One example given by Chalke: a 65-year-old puts $250,000 into a longevity policy today from which s/he can expect to receive as much as $210,000 a year from age 85 on. MetLife has a longevity annuity policy that costs $50,000, and at age 85, pays $35,205 a year for the rest of one's life. If the purchaser dies before 85, it pays nothing. This type of policy might be a good strategy for a healthy, active individual who has a nest egg of two million or more. This retiree could work out a plan whereby both the principal and interest of his/her nest egg could then be spent down over the twenty-year period between 65 and 85, providing the retiree with greater income than s/he would have otherwise had during these same twenty years. Even if the entire nest egg were totally spent down over this 20 year period, this insurance "safety net" would then kick in at age 85 and provide an adequate "forever income."

Avoid Spending on Unnecessary "Luxury" Items

The 1996 book, *The Millionaire Next Door*, should be standard reading material for all doctors. Thomas J. Stanley, Ph.D., and William D. Danko, Ph.D., are the authors who based their results on research data accumulated over a twenty-year period. One startling find of their research pertained specifically to physicians, and this was that, in spite of earning incomes that were more than four times greater than those of the average American household (at the time, $140,000 a year, compared to $33,000), physicians did not tend to accumulate wealth. In fact, compared to all high income producing occupations, the researchers found that physicians had a "significantly low propensity" for accumulating substantial wealth. While there were many reasons given for this finding, it was discovered that it was, in large part, due to the fact that many physician households were concerned with consuming rather than investing – leaving them with little money after funding their high-consumption lifestyles. Because their incomes are typically high, most physicians believe that they can consume now and "make up" the difference later. As is often the case, later never comes – or "later" ends up being a time of recession – which compounds the shortfalls created by bad financial habits.

The authors found seven common denominators amongst those in their study who successfully built wealth. The two most significant were: 1) wealthy people often choose to live well below their means and 2) wealthy people believe that financial independence is more important than displaying a grand social status. Obviously, both of these traits translate into spending less while investing and saving more. Let us examine some examples.

Using the compounding "rule of 72" to estimate the approximate length of time it takes for an investment to double – based on the interest rate, a one time investment of $40,000, compounding each year at a 9% return, would double about every eight years (72 ÷ 9% = 8). If a person were to invest this amount at age 25, it would grow to $1,280,000 by age sixty-five. Many doctors spend at least this amount of $40,000 on a luxury car. Examining this $40,000 car in light of the "rule of 72" puts its real cost at a $1,280,000 loss in savings in the doctor's retirement years. On the other hand, a $7,000 used car would be equivalent to a "loss" of only $224,000 over this same period of time – $1,056,000 less than the more costly alternative. Compounding this effect on future wealth is the fact that many doctors tend to buy several cars at this $40,000 price – or even greater – throughout their careers.

Note also that "small expenses" add up over time. If you were to have one bottle of wine with dinner, the difference between buying a $7 and a $20 bottle would be "just" $13, but if you were to do this every night for one year, this difference would add up to $4,576. Investing this amount each year in a 401K, at an 8% return, would result in $1,185,443 at the end of forty years, with relatively little sacrifice. Keep in mind that for every purchase you make, there are, as in this case, multiple options – including that of foregoing the purchase altogether and investing the money instead.

In her book, entitled, *The Difference: How Anyone Can Prosper in Even the Toughest Times*, the author, Jean Chatzky, estimates that only 3% of the population fits into the financial category of "wealthy." She conducted a survey of 5,000 people and placed each into one of four financial categories. The percentage of the population that fell into each of these categories is shown in *Table 11.4*.

Table 11.4: Financial Categories

Category	Percent in Category
Wealthy	3%
Financially Comfortable	27%
Pay check-to-paycheck	54%
Further-in-debtors	15%

For most physicians, being in the "financially comfortable" group is an achievable goal. Those who feel that they are not in this category, or higher, should take the time to reexamine their financial habits and determine the type of changes they need to make in order to change their situations, especially in the areas of spending and investing. Cutting back should be easier to accomplish during a recession because it is not "cool" to appear "rich" when so many are struggling to make ends meet. Changing financial habits is not something that has to be accomplished overnight, and the changes need not be drastic. Keep in mind that, over time, small changes add up to big results. What is important is that you develop sound financial habits – ones that will serve you well throughout your lifetime.

Own the Home in Which You Live

I recall a patient who retired in 1976. He had purchased his home for $40,000 and sold it for the "outrageous" sum of $120,000, with the intention of renting an apartment and using this real estate profit to support his retirement income. Fifteen years later, this retiree's rent was four times his previous mortgage payment, and his nest egg was barely capable of supporting his profoundly reduced lifestyle. Potential inflation must be accounted for, and its greatest impacts are on home prices, education, health insurance, and the cost of commuting to work. Fortunately, those who are retired, on Medicare, and own their own homes have far less exposure to a cost upturn in any of these segments of the economy. For this reason, I recommend that even if you decide to sell your home, you should utilize some of your equity for retirement and "downsize," still owning the new roof over your head. No one can predict future inflation rates, and home ownership is one of the best protections against inflation because it keeps one of your greatest costs – housing – fixed, regardless of the inflation rate.

One financial "downside" of home ownership may occur during times of recession. This is when home values can decline. The primary protection against this is for those nearing retirement to have relatively small mortgages, or none at all. The closer one gets to retirement, the greater is the investment value of paying down a mortgage. Having a small, or no, mortgage payments serves as the best insurance protecting a retiree from fluctuating real estate values. With little mortgage debt, fluctuation of home prices will be irrelevant to your financial wellbeing, and your lifestyle will be better protected because rent is often a retiree's biggest expense.

Credit Card Fees Can Ruin Retirement Plans

Little is more confusing to the public than credit card fees and interest rates. Most people understand that introductory rates on new cards will increase after a specified period of time and that rates and rules will vary significantly from card to card, but at the time they decide to make a minimum payment on a card, few take the time to determine what the percentage rate will be, and most do not understand the potential card fees and penalties. This is another one of those areas where seemingly small things can add up.

Many consider that making a minimum payment on a credit card is an "easy way" to put off payment on a large amount – believing that this is a good way to conserve money in difficult times and provide them with time to "get back on their feet." In reality, putting off payment creates a problem because minimum payments lower cardholders' monthly outgoes, simultaneously increasing their cash flow and "enabling" them to purchase even more. These purchasers push their balances ever higher – to levels where they are more difficult to pay off.

To get an idea of how high a credit card's interest rate can be, assume that you have a balance of $1,000 on a card, with a minimum payment of $35. At a time when you are short of cash, you might quickly make the decision to pay this minimum, assuming that it will be easier for you to make a larger payment the following month. Even if you decided to discontinue adding new charges to your card in the ensuing months and erase your $1,000 debt by sending in only the minimum each month, you would be sending payments for 49 months – more than four years! The interest in this example translates to an annual rate of 28.93%! It is no wonder that, over time, people acquire huge credit card debt. Because this debt grows so rapidly at these high rates, it could quickly become virtually impossible to pay off. Just imagine the opportunity of receiving an annual return of 28.93% on your investment portfolio. You would double your investment every 2.7 years! The credit card companies are "earning" this level of return on credit card debt.

Even if you handle your credit card debt responsibly and pay off your balance each month, these companies constantly have new tricks up their sleeves, especially when it comes to taking advantage of your children who may not be as financially savvy as you. As an example, my younger daughter was offered a credit card with a $300 limit. We thought it would be a good idea for her to have a card at college for emergencies, and that this would help her build her own credit history. Our one "rule" was that she pay the balance in full, on time, every month. Each time the bill arrived, she *would* pay the full balance – and before the "due" date. She was working under the assumption that because the limit on her card was $300, if she had a statement with charges totaling less than $300 and had sent payment, in full, on time, she would not receive a $35 fee for "exceeding the credit limit," but this additional fee was something which, in practice, she was charged regularly.

As it happened, the end date of the "billing cycle" did not line up with the payment "due" date. After she mailed her payment, and before the company recorded her on-time payment, she would put a new charge on her card which, when added to the amount of the payment she had just "sent in," would "technically" exceed her limit. Because of this, the actual amount she could spend using her credit card, for a period of about a week, was sometimes as little as

$5 or $10. This was, basically, an intended "trap" established by the credit card company to disguise its obscene interest rate as a penalty fee.

When this late fee is recalculated as an interest rate, it becomes extreme because it represents the extension of credit – sometimes for amounts as small as $5 or $10 – for only a few days. For example, if she were to go over her limit by $50 during the period of time that her payment on the balance had not yet been posted to her account, the $35 charge for this additional "$50 loan" would calculate to an interest payment of 70%! It is amazing how fast these "small" amounts add up. While congress has passed laws aimed at curtailing this type of abuse, it is always a good idea to question every fee or penalty charged by a vendor, and it helps to re-calculate any charge as an interest rate in order to fully appreciate its magnitude.

In addition to being aware of potentially outrageous interest rates, you might want to check the service fees and penalties charged by your "friendly bank." In the July 9, 2009 issue of *USA Today*, a representative of the Federal Deposit Insurance Corporation discussed the high cost of "courtesy overdraft" protection extended by many banks, something many doctors turn to for "protection." Overdrafts usually result from an oversight, typically something involving a small amount. According to the article, "If banks cover a $20 charge for insufficient funds with a $27 overdraft fee (the current range for these bank fees is between $22 and $39), this fee would be the equivalent of a 135% interest rate." In order to understand the magnitude of these fees, consider the fact that those receiving them typically pay them within two weeks. If we were to re-calculate this two-week rate as an annual percentage rate, it would technically translate to an annual interest rate of 3,520%. Again, taking the extra step of calculating the implied annual interest rate whenever fees are charged, or penalties levied, puts a different light on their magnitude.

Make Sure You Understand Your Interest Rates

Understanding how interest rates are calculated is important to decisions we will make in both our business and personal lives. One term to be wary of is "simple interest." We should always be on guard when someone mentions the word "simple" in conjunction with "interest" because nothing is actually simple about interest rates. If something is referred to as "simple," a highly educated person may not want to ask for an explanation, feeling that this implies the answer should be "obvious." This facilitates misinterpretation.

My first experience with the term "simple interest" was in the 1970s when my wife and I were looking to purchase a station wagon to accommodate our growing family. The price of the one we selected was $4,500 (cheap by today's standards, yet this was just prior to the double digit inflation of the 70s). At the time, bank interest rates for three-year auto loans were at 7.0%, but the dealer offered us a "better" rate at 6.0%, "simple interest." Financing through the dealer at this "lower rate" seemed to be a no-brainer.

Fortunately, I asked the sales person to walk me through the process of the interest rate's calculation for his dealership's loan. He said the $4,500 total would "simply" be multiplied by 6%, resulting in $270 annual interest ($810 over the three years of the loan). This put the full price of the car at $5,310 ($4,500 + $810 = $5,310), and the monthly payment for this 6% loan, came out to be $147.50. You can imagine my surprise when I realized that this $147.50 monthly payment at 6.0% "simple interest" was higher than the bank's payment of $138.95 at a 7% rate! Over the three years of the loan, the bank's "higher" rate of 7.0% would result in total interest payments of $502.20 ($307.80 less than the dealer's "lower" rate). The discrepancy between these two interest rates lay in the way they were calculated. The bank determined its interest payment monthly, based on that month's unpaid balance, rather than on the total amount borrowed. If the dealer's $147.50 payments had been determined using the same method as the bank, its interest rate, comparatively, would have been 8.755%. Being presented with this information would have made it much "simpler" for me to choose the best loan option because I then would have been able to compare "apples to apples."

There are numerous ways of calculating interest rates, leaving a good deal of room for misinterpretation or for being taken advantage of. Remember this example when you are shopping for a loan, and make sure to determine how the one you are considering is being calculated. Even when you are certain you understand a "deal," always take the time to make comparisons, double check your options, and assure that you are comparing apples to apples. Also, if there are fees or points charged on a loan, be sure to include these before making calculations; otherwise, you will find your total payback higher than expected.

There are numerous examples of situations in which numbers can be "misinterpreted." Sometimes, it is simply a matter of not taking sufficient time to question their meaning, and at others, a vendor has actually made a deliberate attempt to mislead. Either way, it is important that in both your personal and business dealings, you are aware of the potential that numbers have to be misleading – especially percentage rates – even though, at first glance, they may appear to be "simple."

Getting Your Finances Under Control Will Make You Happier

An early casualty of managed care was physician job satisfaction. Admittedly, some doctors were happy practicing medicine in a managed care environment; however, certain factors related to managed care made most of them unhappy, and many attributed this "unhappiness" to declining fees and reduced income. Let us put this income-related "unhappiness" into context. The average mean salary earned by physicians actually ranks the highest amongst 750 occupations, as documented by the US Bureau of Labor Statistics. This might lead us to ask, "What is the relationship between money and happiness?" or, "Will making more money actually make us happier?"

Virtually everything written on the relationship between happiness and money includes the standard disclaimer that "money cannot buy happiness." I believe that most of us would agree with this statement; yet, we also know that there is some tie between the two. Given that happiness is subjective and recognizing that people earning identical incomes experience a wide variation of satisfaction in their lives, I set out to find objective measures of ways in which money is related to the happiness we feel.

I found one objective measure of happiness in a proprietary study funded by *Money Magazine* that was conducted by the market research firm of RoperASW. The researchers interviewed 1,500 Americans, finding that the level of happiness experienced by those interviewed increased as their income increased but that the "happiness curve" for these individuals flattened out when household income reached about $50,000 a year. According to the Bureau of the Census, the median household income at the time of this study was $42,228 – closely approximating the plateau at which additional money earned "bought" little additional happiness. The average physician income is typically stated in terms of *multiples* of this $50,000 mark; so, why are so many physicians unhappy?

Psychology professors Ed Diener of the University of Illinois and Martin E.P. Seligman of the University of Pennsylvania analyzed one hundred fifty studies conducted on the relationship between wealth and happiness. They found that income is an accurate predictor of happiness when moving up the economic ladder from a position of homelessness to one of holding a job that provides enough money for the basic human needs – food, clothing, and shelter. Once an individual earns money beyond what is necessary to cover these basic needs, additional money does not buy "extra" happiness.

These researchers found that in many cases, materialism negatively influenced happiness, and in fact, they found plenty of examples of people who were not living a life of luxury, yet were happy. In their research, Diener and Seligman actually found a much more significant correlation between happiness and matters such as strong social relationships, enjoyable work, a sense of fulfillment, a sense that life has meaning, and active involvement in civic and other groups. While I have no objective data to make the following statement, I would certainly expect that people who are happy in their social relationships, love their jobs, and sense that life has meaning, probably earn above the average of their peers.

The RoperASW researchers found a strong correlation between happiness and "feeling in control of your finances" – a correlation stronger than that between happiness and the amount of money earned above the level of $50,000. In fact, control over finances correlated much more strongly with happiness than did being in control of one's health, friendships, or weight. As a response to these findings, *Money Magazine* outlined the following ten recommendations for gaining greater control over one's money: 1) get "fairly well" organized, 2) pay bills as they come in rather than all at once, 3) keep tabs on your cash, 4) save at least 5% of your household income, 5) protect your family (and yourself), 6) minimize credit-card debt, 7) do unto others, 8) spend sensibly, 9) start working towards your goals, 10) communicate, and 11) attempt not to be consumed with a desire for more. Gaining control of your finances through measures such as these should lead you to greater happiness than a strategy that focuses solely on earning more money.

If all else fails, studies show that people become happier as they age. Recently, the *Proceedings of the National Academies of Science* reported that a downward trend seen in "happiness" during mid-life sharply reverses itself around age 50, and continues to increase as one ages, hitting a peak at age 85. This is good news– especially coupled with the knowledge that if you want to be happier now, you can be proactive, learn ways to gain control of your money, and take the necessary steps to put this knowledge into action.

Epilogue

Effectively running a medical practice in today's high volume, low fee, and highly regulated healthcare environment is an incredibly complex and daunting undertaking. As group size increases, the degree of complexity and opportunity for errors and process breakdowns increase exponentially. Effective management of a medical practice today requires a skill set not taught in medical school. Unfortunately, the full skill set is rarely possessed by the consultants to whom physicians typically turn for advice. A well-run practice requires an understanding of clinical medicine, but the source of the vast majority of cost and quality problems plaguing healthcare today result from faulty decision making and inefficient workflow, rather than from a lack of medical knowledge. Because of this, a doctor's skill set needs to be expanded to include the proven tools taught in *The Medical Practitioner's Survival Handbook* – including an understanding of finance, accounting, economics, operational leverage, economic game theory, industrial engineering, the science of workflow, customer satisfaction, human resource management, appointment scheduling, effective use of technology, group practice dynamics, continuous improvement techniques, practice valuation, negotiating, and management of personal finances. Abdicating management and operational responsibilities to an office manager or CEO does not change the need for this skill set; even employed physicians suffer the consequences of lower quality and lower physician reimbursement that result from poor decision making and inefficient business operations.

Now that you have read *The Medical Practitioner's Survival Handbook*, you should more clearly recognize the problems that plague healthcare in general and your practice specifically. You will see them through a different and more focused lens. Your approach to decision making will be changed forever, and the outcome of your decisions is that you will be led in significantly different, more productive, and exciting directions. As we approach a future where "doing more, with less, and doing it better" is the unequivocal prescription for success, you now possess a rare set of skills needed to write this prescription. If you are not the managing partner or CEO of your group, you will have the skills necessary for evaluating projects *before* they are implemented. My recommendation is that, because many of the subtleties and common sense logic contained within this book can be missed in a first reading, even greater value and a deeper understanding will be obtained upon a second, or even a third, reading.

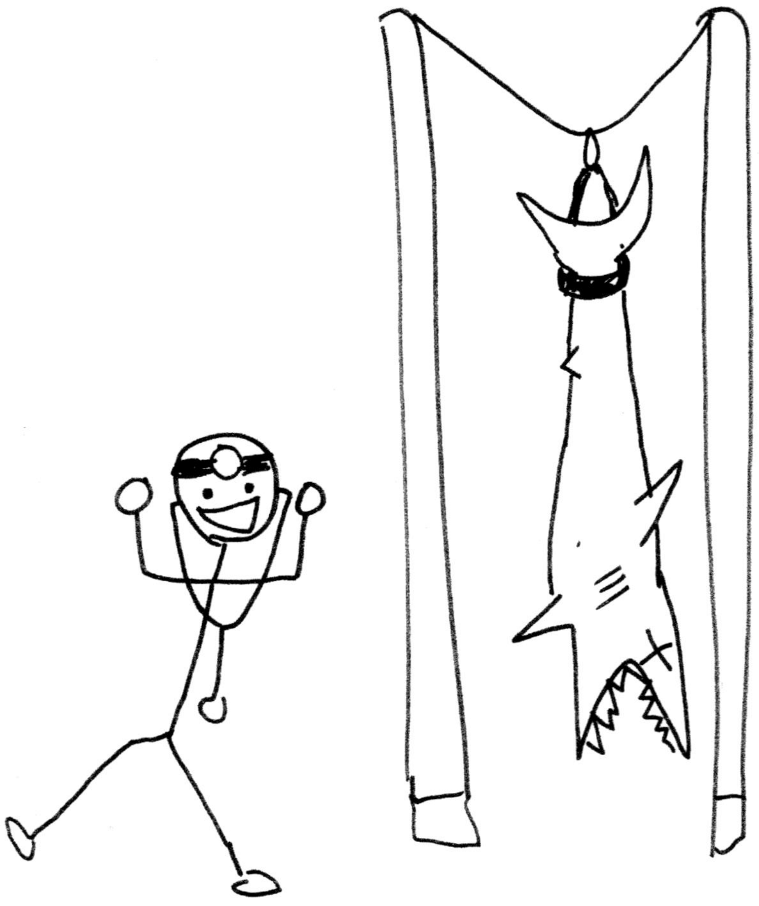